Health Promotion

Praise for the book

The importance of health promotion is currently acknowledged by many health professionals and most politicians; indeed it is frequently equated with public health in general! However, there is at the same time a significant amount of confusion over its definition, meaning and purpose – a situation that is neither helpful for theoreticians and researchers, nor for practitioners. Accordingly this new and accessible book by Kevin Lucas and Barbara Lloyd is a welcome addition to existing texts and makes a refreshing contribution to debate.

While addressing many generally accepted key issues, the authors offer an unorthodox perspective on theory and practice. Unsurprisingly, they challenge the hegemony of the medical model and the narrow individualistic focus on health and its determinants that have been deservedly castigated as 'victim blaming'. They also comment on the occasional sterility of the social cognitive approaches of contemporary health psychology to explaining health choices. However, they do this without the stridency associated with much radical criticism and, more importantly, they invite us to consider – and in some cases rediscover – perspectives on health and health promotion not commonly considered in contemporary texts. They rightly argue that such perspectives may be very fruitful in adding depth and breadth to our understanding of health. In short, Lucas and Lloyd's approach is challenging in its emphasis on a 'positive' and holistic orientation to health and always humane in its emphasis on quality of life and, in the authors' words, 'the indivisibility of the individual from society'.

This new perspective on health promotion complements other key texts in health education and health promotion. I commend it to readers.

Keith Tones

Health Promotion

Evidence and Experience

Kevin Lucas
and
Barbara Lloyd

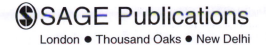
SAGE Publications
London • Thousand Oaks • New Delhi

SAGE Publications Ltd
1 Oliver's Yard
55 City Road
London EC1Y 1SP

SAGE Publications Inc.
2455 Teller Road
Thousand Oaks, California 91320

SAGE Publications India Pvt Ltd
B-42, Panchsheel Enclave
Post Box 4109
New Delhi 110 017

British Library Cataloguing in Publication data

A catalogue record for this book is available from the
British Library

ISBN 0-7619-4005-7
ISBN 0-7619-4006-5 (pbk)

Library of Congress Control Number: 2005901774

Typeset by C&M Digitals (P) Ltd, Chennai, India
Printed on paper from sustainable resources
Printed and bound in Great Britain by Athenaeum Press, Gateshead

Contents

Acknowledgements

We would like to express our gratitude to a number of people who gave their support during the writing of this book, particularly to Helen Lucas, Peter Lloyd and Janet McInnes. Their encouragement is greatly appreciated.

Kevin Lucas and Barbara Lloyd 2005

A personal perspective: Barbara Lloyd

In my early 20s, armed with a bachelor's degree from the University of Chicago and a master's degree in psychology, I spent two years up country in Kenya studying Gusii methods of child-rearing. This fascinating but highly academic research was part of a larger, cross-cultural programme, which posed identical questions about socialisation that had derived from a combination of Freudian and learning theories. So certain were we of the universality of our theoretical approach to an understanding of human development that comparable evidence was collected in India, Mexico, the Philippines, Okinawa and a small town in America.

Five years later I returned to Africa, having completed a PhD at Northwestern University in Illinois; I had gathered survey evidence to test the effects of parental techniques of punishment on the development of children's moral sensibilities. When the Vice-Chancellor of the University of Ibadan questioned me about the usefulness of my rigorous studies of Nigerian child-rearing practices I was flummoxed. I replied that a nation which could fund a vast space programme (my research was supported by a grant from the Ford Foundation) could afford the pursuit of psychological knowledge which was pure and theoretical. Over the years this self-righteous reply has returned to haunt me.

On returning from Nigeria in the mid-1960s I taught developmental-social psychology in academic settings, first at Birmingham University, and then at Sussex. By the 1970s issues of social significance had begun to loom large. It was the second wave of feminism and I was caught up in creating an undergraduate course which would offer first-year students some knowledge of the great debates about the differences between the sexes. Slowly I began to think about the impact of psychological knowledge upon everyday lived experience.

I desired an in-depth understanding of individual development and felt a growing unease with standard evidence-gathering procedures which dictated highly controlled and limited contact with a statistically satisfactory cohort of subjects. This discontent, as well as contemporary theorising about gender, re-wakened an adolescent interest in the writings of Sigmund Freud.

Many strands in my own history were beginning to emerge and to re-order. Using Freudian insights to systematically test hypotheses about the effects of socialisation no longer seemed sufficient. I was not satisfied with observing or testing children on two or three occasions. Piaget, and his followers, could elicit specific answers in order to explain how children came to understand number or space or causality, but Freud dealt with the individual who walked into his consulting room. It seemed important to encounter people over months or even years in order to appreciate their individuality. I wanted to understand the whole person, and thus I trained as a psychoanalytic psychotherapist.

For many years I kept these two strands quite separate. I taught and gathered evidence in orthodox ways within the university, and tried equally to maintain the frame of professional rigor in my analytic encounters. It seemed that evidence and experience were forever separated. Things began to change in the late 1980s when I directed a study which sought to evaluate the effects on infants of living with their mothers in HM prisons in mother/baby units. Shortly after that I became involved in the supervision of Kevin's doctoral research on smoking in pregnancy. We both voiced doubts about the limits which his rigorous data collection imposed upon an understanding of women's smoking behaviour while they were pregnant.

In 1990 I took early retirement at Sussex University and then spent the next 12 years working with Kevin on research in which we have attempted to employ methods which would impose less and tell us more about the individuals we were studying. My reputation in the field of gender studies and Kevin's systematic research on smoking led to a substantial research grant from the Department of Health aimed at understanding gender differences in adolescents' smoking experiences. This research gave us the opportunity to bring together our interest in experience as well as in systematic survey evidence.

Freedom from the standard academic activities of teaching and administration enabled me to develop my clinical practice as a psychoanalytic psychotherapist and to read more widely in that field. It has led me to explore at length a new tradition within psychoanalysis, the relational approach. I have found Jessica Benjamin's (1998) concern with the developmental importance of the capacity to recognise other subjects a bridge which may help to bring evidence and experience closer together.

A personal perspective: Kevin Lucas

I initially trained as a psychiatric nurse in 1973. At that time, much of psychiatric practice took place in large mental hospitals, generally sited in isolated, rural locations. My experience was typical of the time. The institution stood in several hundred acres of its own grounds, comprising a mixture of park, farm and woodland, and housed over one thousand patients. In addition, it employed hundreds of people, many of whom were resident in accommodation in the grounds, with nearly all the rest living in a small market town about a mile away; for many years, the hospital was by far the town's most important employer. The hospital had its own farm, kitchen gardens and a small army of trades people, making it not unlike a rural village in its own right.

Ironically, there were actually certain advantages to this arrangement for those cared for in such an environment, which sadly cannot be assumed for people with mental health problems today: reliable accommodation, regular meals, adequate clothing and swift and easy access to nursing and medical care, combined with a relative immunity to the penalties that the current criminal justice system imposes in response to some of the manifestations of mental illness. Yet there were overwhelming disadvantages. While efficient in delivering such basic aspects of care, the system denied many people some of the most fundamental rights of dignity, independence, individuality and self-determination. Moreover, the identities of so-called 'psychiatric patients' were defined primarily by their illnesses, rather than their unique characteristics as people. It seemed that despite meeting some of the needs of our patients, many of the everyday social interactions, opportunities for companionship and activities which make life meaningful and provide a sense of identity and belonging were simply not considered in planning and delivering their care.

Later, I spent several years working in an acute general hospital where, despite the very best of intentions, somewhat analogous processes of dehumanisation appeared to take place. Of course, we never saw it that way at the time; we prided ourselves on our clinical expertise and ability to treat illness and alleviate pain. Yet even then, nurses and doctors who were able to treat their patients as whole human beings, rather than 'cases', were less commonplace than one might expect. Those who did stood out and their example has helped inform this book.

My dissatisfaction with such issues led to my undertaking a series of academic endeavours. Following a first degree in the natural sciences, I undertook a postgraduate course in health promotion at what was, at that time, considered to be something of a 'radical polytechnic'. There, I became inspired by the way in which traditional, medicalised notions of health and disease could be challenged. During a subsequent decade of working in health promotion in the NHS an interest in research grew, resulting in a PhD in health psychology some 12 years ago.

More latterly, as a full-time academic, I am aware of the enormous pressures for us to further our disciplines and for such advances to result in publications. But I also believe that another, complementary, approach is needed on which to develop health promotion activity. Both my own everyday observations and my empirical research have led me to the conclusion that there is something fundamentally lacking in the way that health promotion is planned, prioritised, operationalised and evaluated, at least in the UK.

It was at that point that it became clear that Barbara Lloyd and I had reached very similar conclusions, despite having come from what might be described as opposite histories. I had spent many years in the NHS working in clinical, health promotion and public health settings, before entering academia. Conversely, Barbara had spent many years as an academic psychologist and psychotherapist, before becoming involved in our joint research in health promotion.

The result of this mirror-image of evidence and experience is this book. In it, we propose a particular point of view. This view is balanced, as best we are able, but we are aware that we may risk some readers finding our approach somewhat polemical. In our early discussions with Sage, we had proposed the title *The Emperor's New Clothes*, but our commissioning editor wisely advised against such a notion. Yet we still believe that there is much evidence available which is given less attention by health promotion planners than should be the case. We also believe very strongly that there are alternative approaches to health promotion that are worthy of serious consideration. For this reason, we have expressed our views, and those of many others in the field, in a direct manner. Yet our intention is not to offend, nor to challenge the need for many of the activities carried out by health promotion workers, nor even to be critical in a negative sense. What we hope to achieve in this book is to provide a focused starting point for debate as to how health promotion might be broadened in scope, and perhaps be made more effective in the complex social environment of 21st-century Britain.

ONE   Health and health promotion: 'Theory', models and approaches

A little experience often upsets a lot of theory.

S. Parkes Cadman

Introduction

In this opening chapter, we outline some of the most influential (and most contested) definitions of health, and approaches to health promotion. Although some success has been claimed for health promotion interventions, in general the results to date have been modest: for example, safer sex campaigns in preventing HIV infection among gay men. In other areas efforts have been remarkably disappointing, notably in preventing smoking uptake among adolescents. 'Health promotion' is a term which has been applied to a very wide range of activities performed in many and diverse contexts. Often there has been little regard for whether the ways in which professionals would like to improve other people's health is the way that those *people feel is important for themselves*. Perhaps this failure to match the goals of professionals to the health concerns of ordinary people accounts for these uneven results. We believe that this mismatch is significant and it is from this perspective that we have approached this book.

'Theory'

In our combined 40-odd years' experience of working with health promotion practitioners, both 'specialist' (such as health promotion advisers and public health doctors) and others whose activities involve more direct contact with the public (such as teachers, health visitors, nurses and other health professionals), we have found that, in practice, the terms 'theory', 'model', 'evidence' and 'approach' are often used interchangeably. Perhaps one reason for this stems from the multidisciplinary nature of contributions to the health promotion literature. For example, medical practitioners might consider 'evidence' to be provided by data on therapeutic levels of drugs or vaccines. By contrast, some health psychologists propose that 'evidence-based health promotion' may be provided by using sophisticated statistical techniques to identify variables which (assuming they can be manipulated) might influence behaviour. Health promotion workers, on the other hand, often consider the existence of a theoretical model to support an intervention as constituting 'evidence' of how it should be implemented.

Although many academic writers will (perhaps rightly) consider such a lack of precision to be intellectually slapdash, it is easy to understand why, in practical terms, it is useful: *all are attempts to guide health promotion activity by some kind of rationale*. In this chapter, we, therefore, are guilty of the same laxity. *We employ the term 'Theory' here to mean any kind of theory, model, approach or empirical evidence which is employed to provide a rationale for the planning, operationalisation or subsequent evaluation of health promotion activities.*

Because of the widely differing social, political and technological circumstances worldwide, this volume addresses itself principally to health promotion activity in the UK. In a recent, concise yet comprehensive overview of health promotion theory, Nutbeam and Harris (2004) also adopt such a pragmatic approach. The latter part of this chapter draws on their analysis and seeks to place recent developments in health promotion within a UK framework.

Defining health

Before embarking on health promotion activity, it is essential to identify what should be the target for change. In order to do this, it is necessary to have a clear understanding of what 'health' is before we can begin to set about 'promoting', 'improving' or (to use the currently fashionable term) 'developing' it. Despite being nearly 60 years old, it is still worth starting from the World Health Organization's (WHO) definition of health as 'a state of complete physical, mental and social well-being and not merely the absence of disease'. Of course, this notion of health is impossibly idealistic and unobtainable for just about anybody. Moreover, it suggests that anyone with the slightest imperfection in their bodily, psychological or social functioning cannot be 'healthy'. Yet this much-criticised, utopian and somewhat dated notion is still a worthy platform for a discussion of what 'health' might be. For at its heart, the idea that health might be something other than the absence of disease was a fundamental shift in mainstream thought in the 1940s, and one to which we will return repeatedly in this book when considering current health promotion activity in the UK.

A different view of health was proposed some 30 years later by Talcott Parsons (1972). Parsons suggested that health might be seen as 'the state of optimum capacity of an individual for the effective performance of the roles and tasks for which (s)he has been socialised' (p. 117). Like the WHO's definition, this concept may be criticised for being too idealistic. Moreover, such a definition implies that the primary value of an individual's health is that she or he can perform the tasks expected of them in society. While such a view might be attractive to some politicians, it tends to minimise the importance of *quality* of life as being a legitimate goal in its own right. 'Quality of life' is a complex concept and is not easy to define. It is certainly not the preserve of the fit, well and healthy envisaged by the WHO. A comprehensive account of the nature and factors which contribute to the quality of life among those who are chronically ill is beyond the scope of this volume, but is provided in exemplary fashion by Fallowfield (1990). She illustrates the need to consider quality of life as a primary aim for health professionals working with people who have cancers, AIDS, cardiovascular diseases, arthritis, with elderly people and people who are dying.

Many other definitions of health, with varying degrees of usefulness, have been presented, but one lasting notion is that health is a form of commodity which can be 'bought' and 'sold', either metaphorically or literally. As Seedhouse (1986) suggests, health is often viewed as a commodity, 'that it is something – albeit an amorphous thing – which can be supplied. Equally, it is something which can be lost'(p. 34). As Aggleton (1994) points out, it follows from this perspective that health can be bought by investing in private health care, sold via health food shops, given by drugs or surgery, and lost by accidents or disease. It is not difficult to appreciate the connection between such ideas and the development of modern medicine within the uncontrolled commercial environment of the late 20th century.

A further concept of health, and one which has been adopted enthusiastically by health promoters in the past, is that of achieving personal potential. Here, health is seen as being composed of a number of 'factors' which enable, or at least help, people to achieve all that they have the potential to become. Such notions were employed explicitly in some health promotion campaigns of the 1980s and 1990s which commonly used 'Be All You Can Be!' and similar phrases as straplines in a range of initiatives (for example, HEBS, 1998). Seedhouse (1986) describes these factors, present in each individual in a unique combination, as 'foundations for achievement'. However, proponents of this concept of health generally offer little theory-based guidance on what such factors might be or how they might combine to produce potential, which itself is not always clearly defined. Aggleton (1994) is dismissive of 'achieving personal potential' as a means of defining health on the grounds that it 'remains a little mystical, perhaps no more easily attainable than the state of complete mental, physical and social well being that the WHO talked about in 1946' (p. 12).

The diverse definitions of health we have presented so far share one characteristic in common: they are all definitions provided by academics, whether as individuals or as collectives. Perhaps more germane to this volume are ideas about the nature of health that are held by the people who are the intended targets of health promotion activity: that is, lay concepts of the nature of health and disease, or how 'ordinary people' perceive their own health and what is important to them. Over 30 years ago, Herzlich (1973) demonstrated clearly that lay people distinguish much more sharply between health and illness than many health professionals (at least in our experience) habitually do, and this is still true, even today. In a sample of French, predominantly middle-class subjects, Herzlich's respondents identified health as being not only the absence of disease, but also as a reserve of well-being, individually determined by constitution and temperament as well as a positive state of equilibrium.

Similar lay definitions of health have been variously described by Pill and Stott (1982), Blaxter and Paterson (1982), Williams (1983) and Blaxter (1985). Blaxter (1983) reported that lay people also view health in terms of will-power, self-discipline, and self-control, qualities consistent with the notion among both industrialised and developing societies that one has a duty to be well, and that being ill carries some suggestion of failure.

However, it would be an over-simplification to suggest that all lay people hold similar views as to the nature of health. Some studies have suggested that social class influences how health is perceived. For example, d'Houtard and Field (1984) found that middle-class respondents were more likely to define health in positive terms such as 'fitness' than were their working-class contemporaries. Conversely, Calnan (1987) found a less pronounced difference, and points out that variations found in responses may be related to differences in education. Nevertheless, if given adequate time, relatively poorly-educated respondents are able to express very complex ideas about the nature of health (Blaxter, 1983; Cornwell, 1984).

More recently Blaxter (1995a) conducted a survey with a large sample, in which she explored lay people's beliefs about disease and other aspects of illness, and also asked questions about what they considered health to be, both for themselves and for others.

Firstly, respondents were asked to think of someone they knew who was very healthy, and asked *what made them call that person 'healthy'*.

Secondly, respondents were asked to describe what it was like *when they were healthy*. Blaxter identified eight major categories of response to these questions:

Health as not being ill

Using this definition of health, respondents were more likely to describe themselves as healthy because of an absence of specific symptoms, while never or rarely attending a doctor was more commonly seen as 'proof' of the health of others. In contrast to d'Houtard and Field's (1984) earlier work, Blaxter found little evidence that such definitions were used more by less affluent respondents, and she attributes this difference to the small sample size employed in the earlier study. Interestingly, less than half as many men who had a chronic illness used this definition compared to men who did not have such an illness. Blaxter concludes that 'if illness symptoms are a taken for granted experience, or disease is seen as the norm, then health has to be defined in other ways' (1995a: 22).

Health as a reserve

Here, a person is seen as healthy because they recover quickly from illness, as a result of having a 'reserve' of health on which to call. Occasionally, this is seen as inborn or inherited.

Health as behaviour

Frequently, Blaxter's respondents described health in terms of 'virtuous behaviours', including regular exercise, a healthy diet, non-smoking and moderate alcohol use. However, Blaxter notes that this kind of response was particularly prevalent among younger, less-educated individuals who may simply have found describing health too difficult a task, preferring to answer the somewhat simpler question 'what makes them healthy' to 'what makes you call them healthy'. Yet the manner in which these ideas were expressed led Blaxter to believe that, for some individuals, 'health was identical with the healthy life'. Although they could offer no evidence for their chosen person's health status, it was simply assumed that one adopting such a lifestyle must necessarily be healthy.

Health as physical fitness

Some of Blaxter's respondents defined health in terms of physical fitness. Unsurprisingly, such responses were more common among younger respondents, and also among men. The person respondents chose to describe was very likely to be male, with 80% of men using this description identifying a man, and 57% of women using this description also identifying men as subjects.

Health as energy or vitality

'Energy' was the word most commonly used by older men and all women when describing health, and was used almost as frequently by young men as 'fitness'. Although sometimes physical energy was being described, often respondents referred to a kind of psychosocial vitality unrelated to physical activity, using terms such as 'lively', 'alert' and being 'keen and interested' or 'full of life'. These descriptions were often in the context of work and feelings of enthusiasm for it.

Health as social relationships

Women were much more likely than were men to define their own health in terms of their relationships with other people. Many women mentioned their families in their definitions of health for themselves: 'coping with the family', 'enjoying the family' and 'having more patience with them' were common responses among younger women. Being in a position to help or to care for others was often cited by older women; the willingness and ability to help people was also a very common response among older women when describing other people's health as well as their own.

Health as function

For some people, health was seen as being able to do the thing that they needed to be able to do. While some respondents described this in terms of being able to do their work, others spoke of being able to look after members of their families. Clearly, this category has overlap with the previous two described, but Blaxter distinguishes them by the functional emphasis of these types of responses: being able to respond to whatever demands happen to present themselves during everyday life.

Health as psychosocial well-being

Blaxter's final category of lay descriptions of health concerns issues that, we believe, should be the focus of much more health promotion activity (and funding) than is currently the case. *Despite careful coding to exclude descriptions which could be classified in other categories, this category of description was the one most commonly used by all subjects who were middle-aged and older.* In addition, 10% of the whole sample used expressions such as 'enjoys life' in their descriptors of 'someone who is very healthy'. Blaxter's respondents' descriptions of 'psychosocial well-being' are both complex and far-reaching. For some respondents, an explicitly holistic view of health was used:

> She's a person with a spiritual core. She's physically, mentally and spiritually as one.

For others, terms describing confidence and pride were common:

> health is to feel proud – when you can go out and you can hold your head up, look good. You don't have so many hang-ups and you can think straight.

Some of the most common phrases used were 'living life to the full', 'happy to be alive'. Some respondents defined their own health in terms of their contentment with their world:

> Well, I think health is when you feel happy. Because I know when I'm happy I feel quite well.

> I've reached the stage now where I say isn't it lovely and good to be alive … it's wonderful to be alive and to be able to stand and stare!

It is interesting to note at this point that these two descriptors were provided by respondents who were both in their 70s. Although Blaxter's description does not specifically identify the physical health status of these two respondents, we note that their choice of 'psychosocial well-being' descriptors are those concerned with physical functioning; this is in marked contrast to the descriptors used by the youngest section of the sample who might be expected to have fewer physical disabilities. Moreover, many respondents described their own health as 'excellent' when this was clearly not the case in purely physical terms. It is also worth bearing in mind that Blaxter's respondents' self-assessments showed trends with social class, geographic region and deprivation indicators that are wholly consistent with socio-economic trends with morbidity discussed in Chapter 3.

In Blaxter's sample, this difference in the ways in which lay people describe their own and others' health showed a distinct pattern through the life course. Younger men tended to use descriptors indicating physical fitness and strength, and often named athletes as examples of healthy others. Middle-aged and older people, especially women, expressed much more complex ideas of what health was for themselves and for other people, with emphasis on psychosocial issues as described above, including the importance of social relationships in assessing their own state of health.

Defining health promotion

Arguably, the most influential single volume on health promotion practice in the UK has been Linda Ewles and Ina Simnett's *Promoting Health*, originally published in 1985 and still a standard text for health promotion students and health professionals 20 years later. They have expanded the WHO's definition of health to include emotional, spiritual and societal aspects of health. Ewles and Simnett propose six areas of human existence in which health may be considered:

- Physical health: concerned with the mechanistic functioning of the body
- Mental health: concerned with the ability to think clearly and coherently
- Emotional or affective health: the ability to recognise and express emotions appropriately and to cope with stress, depression and anxiety
- Social health: the ability to make and maintain relationships
- Spiritual health: either related to religious beliefs and practices, or with ways of achieving peace of mind
- Societal health: concerned with the capacity of the society in which an individual lives, which supplies the human needs of freedom and opportunity as well as the basic infrastructure for them to be exercised.

Other writers have extended Ewles and Simnett's list even further. For example, Aggleton and Homans (1987) suggest that in addition to these six categories, it is also necessary to consider a person's sensual and sexual health.

Much of this book is concerned with the last four of Ewles and Simnett's categories. *We believe that if 'health' is to mean anything beyond the absence or cure of disease, then 'health promotion' should have as its primary foci of activity the emotional, social, spiritual and societal aspects of everyday life.*

For several decades, programmes designed to improve people's health have been based, either explicitly or more loosely, on a number of influential social psychological models. The reasoning underlying the adoption of these theories has been that if factors that predict health-related behaviour can be identified, then modifying these factors in some way is likely to bring about behavioural change, preferably from unhealthy to healthier habits. The success of initiatives based on these models has been mixed; critique of such models and explanations is the subject of Chapter 5 of this book.

In this first chapter, however, we will examine primarily those ideas which seek to improve health by bringing about changes in communities, rather than those which attempt to modify individual behaviours by employing a sophisticated model of individual choice.

For example, the target of a proposed intervention may be altering socially-accepted norms. Such approaches may be argued as having produced results: public attitudes towards drink-driving, and the wearing of seatbelts provide good examples. Roadside breath-testing and legislation requiring the use of seatbelts in the front of vehicles were both met with popular opposition and criticism when first introduced, yet today drink-driving is rightly viewed as criminally irresponsible; similarly, an individual who is injured in a road traffic accident as a result of failure to wear a seatbelt is likely to be seen as foolhardy rather than worthy of sympathy.

Similarly, the target of health promotion activity may be change in organisational practices. For example, stress-reduction and anti-bullying policies are now routine elements of human resource activity throughout public sector employment in a way unimaginable 30 years ago, when intimidation in the workplace went largely unchallenged. In both these examples, health promotion theory has been derived from the knowledge base of the particular disciplines involved, namely social psychology and corporate management. Theory is also valuable in planning solutions to identified problems. In the human resources example above, theory helps to identify where change can be made, and what elements of policy will be necessary to achieve the objectives specified.

Perhaps the simplest means of attempting to bring about a change in social norms is by communicating messages about how people 'should' behave. Theory concerning effective communication on a large scale has been used to shape 'public education' campaigns for many years. In order for changes in social norms to be achieved, communities need to understand why a particular issue is sufficiently important that values different to their current ones should be adopted. In short, ideas about changing health-related behaviours need to be 'marketed'. The application of commercial marketing theory to health promotion has a history of over 30 years; this adaptation has been termed social marketing (Maibach et al., 2002). It has also recently become explicit in government policy, as described later in this chapter.

Using marketing terminology, Maibach and colleagues suggest that health promoters need to understand the perceived interest of 'target market members', to 'enhance and deliver the package of benefits associated with a product, service or idea', and to 'reduce the barriers that interfere with the adoption or maintenance of that product, service or idea'. Thus 'market members' (the target groups of a health promotion campaign) 'expend resources' (for example, time, effort or willpower) when the product (behaviour) on offer provides clear advantages over their current state or practices (improved health). Thus the 'product' may be smoking cessation, which carries attractive benefits in terms of risk reduction, financial savings and personal attractiveness, weighed against perceived stress reduction, creation of personal space and other benefits smokers commonly report as a result of smoking. Provided non-smoking can be seen as accruing more advantages than smoking, it is suggested that that option will become attractive to more and more individuals until it is seen as a generally socially preferable norm.

The process of social marketing has a series of stages: marketing analysis, which requires an appreciation of current attitudes, knowledge and practices. This allows for the planning of interventions for specific target groups. Once the needs and interests of the target group have been identified, consideration is given to the materials to be employed in the campaign. Paper-based resources such as leaflets, flyers and other materials are designed with the characteristics of the target group as a focus. Publicity may be sought by many means such as advertising, news media coverage, sponsorship, endorsement by famous individuals who are thought likely to be influential on the target group (for example, footballers and pop musicians are often chosen when seeking to influence young people) or competitions with prizes. The final consideration in marketing is placement: how the product can be accessed by the intended 'consumers'; in the case of smoking cessation, this will involve where would-be ex-smokers can obtain nicotine replacement preparations or access support from suitably-trained professionals.

A good example of these processes may be seen in the operationalisation of the UK's No Smoking Day, an annual event since the early 1980s, in which a series of different groups have been targeted over the years that the campaign has been run. As all successful marketing enterprises contribute to changes in public opinion or behaviour, the successful changes have to be incorporated into the campaign the next time around. Messages employed also change over time to reflect changes in public attitudes, behaviours and ultimately social norms.

While some health promoters might baulk at the commercial language employed in social marketing, the principles expounded are quite consistent with more familiar health promotion theory, such as the decisional balance described by the Health Belief Model (see Chapter 5). Norms are a variable in the Health Belief Model, and are a concept that social psychology has borrowed from sociology.

In examining how theory may influence the development of health promotion programmes aimed at communities, rather than individuals, it is helpful to be clear about what a 'community' may be. In this context, Nutbeam and Harris (2004) consider communities to be defined as: 'dynamic systems with inherent strengths and capabilities that can be influenced and supported in ways that will improve health' (p. 25).

This definition is useful as it sets out the key assumptions made in attempts to improve the health of a community:

- that the community has the latent potential for improved health
- that this potential can be realised by intervention.

Clearly, communities with the greatest potential for improved health are those which are also the least healthy (and often the most materially deprived). Nutbeam and Harris cite the work of Rogers (1983; 2002) which ably describes the processes and nature of how 'innovation', or changes, may permeate through a community. Rogers suggests that different individuals adopt new ideas (for example, concerning health-related behaviours such as smoking, diet or exercise) with different degrees of ease or difficulty, and hence behavioural changes occur at different rates among different groups in a community. Rogers identifies five such groups:

- **Innovators**: those individuals who are first to assimilate new ideas and respond to them, estimated to be around 2–3% of the population
- **Early adopters**: those individuals who, though less immediately responsive than the innovators, are nevertheless quick to respond to new ideas, not least because they possess the financial and other attributes necessary to do so, estimated to be around 10–15% of the population
- **Early majority**: this larger group is next to adopt changes in behaviour consistent with the new idea; Rogers estimates them to represent 30–35% of the population
- **Late majority**: this group tend to be less open to the new idea. More sceptical than the others, they modify their behaviour only when any associated benefits are firmly demonstrated. They may constitute around 30–35% of the population
- **Laggards**: this group is the slowest to respond to new ideas and may actively resist change; they represent the remaining 1–20% of the population.

For those charged with planning health promotion activities, the relevance of Rogers' classification is obvious: it is critical to understand which section of the community is being targeted in order that the design, nature and delivery of the initiative are appropriate to that particular group. Many factors are likely to determine into which of Rogers' categories an individual may fall, but (in the UK at least) the most influential are probably social class, age, education, disposable income, as well as ethnicity and/or religious affiliation. In addition, the nature of the innovation is likely to influence the speed at which it is adopted: the greater or more radical the change, the greater the resistance is likely to be.

The manner in which an intervention is operationalised will also influence the rate of its adoption. Legislative measures (for example, seatbelt use in cars to reduce the incidence of injuries) have brought about a far swifter adoption of behavioural change, even among the Late Majority and Laggards than have some more recent attempts to change behaviour based primarily on information-giving (for example, 'sun-safety' campaigns which aim to reduce the incidence of skin cancer).

In approaches to health promotion which aim to influence communities, the function of the health promotion worker differs depending on the particular strategy adopted. Citing a typology developed by Rothman (2001), Nutbeam and Harris (2004) describe three ways of working with communities whose principles underpin health promotion interventions:

- **Locality development**: this approach encourages community participation and the involvement of people in addressing the everyday problems which they collectively face. The health promoter's task is to facilitate co-operation between individuals: to work as a catalyst to enable changes to be made, rather than to initiate or direct change.
- **Social planning**: in this approach, the health promoter's task is to gather data regarding the health needs of the community and to plan ways in which these may be addressed. Generally based on epidemiological analyses of illness, priorities are determined by, and the programmes delivered through, experts and professionals.
- **Social action**: this approach focuses on the most disadvantaged members of a community and the health promoter's task is one of advocacy to enable disempowered individuals and groups, a process often described as 'building community capacity'.

Despite providing useful notions of how health promotion activities might be structured within communities, Rothman's concepts have their limitations: firstly, they may be seen as being focused too exclusively on the solving of specific, pre-defined 'problems', rather than representing ways of improving health status generally. This is an important consideration: as Hawe et al. (2000) have pointed out, there is 'little value in building a system that cements in today's solution to today's problems. We need to create a more innovative capability so that in the future the system or community we are working with can respond appropriately to new problems in unfamiliar contexts' (p. 3). Secondly, some health promoters see such methods as being too dependent on 'expert' and professional input. Moreover, Hawe et al. (2000) describe capacity-building as having become 'something of a buzz-word in health promotion practice ... in wider arenas'.

A particularly useful attempt to bring clarity and rigour to the planning, implementation and evaluation of community-based health promotion programmes is found in the work of Bush, Dower and Mutch (2002). Based at the University of Queensland, Bush and colleagues have attempted to measure community capacity by developing an instrument known as the Community Capacity Index (CCI). The CCI is a tool designed to help identify the extent of existing capacity available within a network of organisations and groups at the local level. The aim of the CCI is to gather evidence about the capacity of a network, and then to map that evidence against a set of indicators. In this way, the CCI may be used to set out or to clarify capacity-building as a concept, but equally importantly as a means of evaluating attempts to develop it.

The CCI examines capacity across four domains, namely:

- **Network partnerships**: whether there is capacity to identify the organisations and groups with resources to implement and sustain a programme, whether there is a capacity to deliver the programme, and whether there is a sustainable network established to maintain and resource the programme. It questions whether, and to what degree, all groups and organisations important in the community in question are involved with the work.
- **Knowledge transfer**: whether there is the capacity to transfer knowledge in order to achieve the desired outcomes, as well as to integrate a programme into the mainstream practices of the network partners identified above.
- **Problem solving**: whether there is the capacity within the community or its networks to identify and overcome problems which may be encountered in achieving the desired outcomes.
- **Infrastructure**: whether there is sufficient investment – financial, intellectual and human – made by the network members in order for the programme to be sustainable.

At this point, it is important to emphasise that, by their nature, these *focus on those issues identified by the communities themselves*. It follows, therefore, that issues identified as being important by communities themselves may differ from those that 'experts' (for example, public health doctors and epidemiologists) identify for them. As Nutbeam and Harris (2004) note:

> When thinking about working in and with communities it is important that practitioners reflect on the extent to which their work is focused on problems that have been identified by the community ... service providers may decide that the biggest issue in a community is coronary heart disease, while the community itself may be more concerned with the high levels of crime in the area. Negotiating these different perspectives will be important in planning effective action. (p. 34)

Moreover, despite being an attractive concept, community building is very difficult to achieve in practice. It requires professionals to understand and *accept as valid* values which may be different from their own, especially if the latter are based on epidemiological evidence and used to drive morbidity and mortality reduction 'targets' which, as government employed health promoters, they are expected to achieve. The tension between what 'ordinary people' perceive as being effective in improving the quality of their lives and experts' desire to reduce the incidence of disease (and politicians' desire to reduce the costs of treating it) is a theme which runs throughout this volume. Moreover, community building approaches are often intended to help the most disadvantaged individuals and groups in society, whose marginalisation may result in 'communities' which are weakly identifiable in social terms and physically transient in nature.

Nevertheless, attempts to base community projects on some form of rationale are laudable, and often in ironic contrast to some situations in the public sector, where most professional health promoters are employed. Within British health and social services, it is widely accepted as axiomatic that collaboration between statutory, voluntary and commercial agencies is vital to take health promotion forward. As a result, 'partnerships', 'collaboration' and 'working together' are terms found scattered liberally throughout the documentation of health promotion planning over the last 10 years or so. At first sight, such principles are entirely consistent with a discipline that has long recognised the fact that improving people's health is an aim that cannot be achieved from within health services alone. It is self-evident that lasting benefits to health can only be obtained by co-operation between all statutory bodies, together with voluntary, community and commercial groups. Yet as Nutbeam and Harris (2004) point out:

> there is increasing concern that the level of investment that is required in establishing and maintaining effective relationships may be greater than the benefits. For this reason it is important to develop a critical approach to deciding if, and how, these relationships should be developed and what it is that we hope will be achieved by them. (p. 58)

It might be reasonable, therefore, to expect that Theory might also help to guide the building of professional partnerships which may be necessary to improve health. Regrettably, theoretical explanations of precisely *how* the recent plethora of such partnerships will bring about improvements in the health and well-being of the most vulnerable are far less common than are exhortations to form them. An example of this uncertainty is provided by a recent job advertisement for a health promotion post, which we have anonymised and reproduced below:

Health Improvement Co-ordinator

Primary Care Trust works closely with a range of partners across the ... and ... district council areas to lead the facilitation of the joint ... and ... Health Improvement Partnership.

This is a well-established partnership that ensures the implementation of work plans that respond to identified local priorities, as well as informing the work of the local strategic partnerships and contributing to meeting PCT targets to improve the health and well being of our local populations.

This new role has been developed to provide some dedicated support to the partnership to carry out this work. You will facilitate the development of the partnership's programme, help monitor its progress and support the process of agreeing performance indicators.

You will work across both ... and ... district areas with a range of agencies, to ensure that evidence-based, targeted action is taken to support the health improvement agenda.

Experience of partnership working is essential, together with an understanding of health improvement and equity.

Such paucity of Theory is particularly prevalent in the area of developing healthy public policies. For many years, there has been a growing recognition that many, perhaps most, of the determinants of an individual's health status may not be within their personal control. Relative poverty, poor housing, inadequate education, unemployment and social exclusion combine to render many people's health and life expectancy far poorer than their more affluent and educated contemporaries, who possess all the material resources and opportunities that accompany financial security and sought-after skills.

It follows that if policies which address issues such as housing, training and employment can be developed, they have the potential to improve health, particularly that of the most disempowered and vulnerable members of our society. For this reason, 'developing health public policy' has been an area of health promotion which has received much recent attention. Nutbeam and Harris (2004) describe it as 'still a developing area in health promotion' and they rightly observe that 'even the most casual observer of health public policy can see that there is often a poor relationship between factors that cause or could prevent illness and disability and the policies in place about these issues'. (p. 64)

Nevertheless, they do cite the innovative work of Weiss (1979), who has proposed a collection of five models to illustrate different way in which evidence may guide policy-making aimed at improving health. The first three of these models suggest positive ways in which evidence can be used to inform policy-making, and the remaining two are a more critical assessment of the role of evidence in the development of public policy. Firstly, she proposes a *knowledge-driven* model, in which research findings automatically create a pressure for application in public policy because human benefits can be clearly seen, even if cost-benefit analyses have not yet been calculated. Secondly, a *problem-solving* model can provide a starting point for policy development, based on reviews of available evidence. However, such a model assumes a rational, iterative process to policy-making and effective mechanisms by which evidence from disparate sources can be efficiently gathered and presented to policy-makers. Thirdly, Weiss suggests an *interactive* model in which past experience, political insights and social pressures contribute to the policy-making process in combination with research findings.

More sinisterly, a *political* model of health policy-making can be seen to operate when research findings are used to justify pre-existing or pre-determined positions. Such selective and misrepresentative use of data may be employed to justify current health promotion activity, even if it is ineffective. Nutbeam and Harris (2004) suggest that the exclusive use of mass-media campaigns and school-based interventions to address complex and multifactorial issues such as drug misuse can be interpreted as examples of this model. Certainly, the history of health promotion campaigns in the UK contains many examples of the oversimplification of research data to provide unequivocal messages for a mass audience (for example, see Davison et al., 1991), and this theme is explored in Chapter 2. Finally, Weiss suggests that a *tactical* model is employed by policy-makers when trying to delay making a decision, or to avoid taking responsibility for a decision likely to be unpopular. In contrast to the *political* model in which selective research findings are employed with great certainty, a *tactical* approach actively exploits the normal uncertainty associated with research findings and statistical analyses, claiming that a decision must be delayed until 'more evidence is gathered'. We believe that such a model is likely to be familiar to most casual observers of policy-making in the UK.

Despite this latter pessimistic observation, more recent developments in the application of evidence to health policy-making have emerged. Probably the most influential of these is the concept of a health impact assessment (HIA).

HIAs set out to predict the likely effect a health promotion proposal might have on the health of a given population. Target population may be defined in terms of a geographical area, or a particular group of people sharing a given characteristic such as age, ethnicity, or social class. While this might seem an obvious starting point for any health promotion initiative, the value of assessing impact formally may lie in ensuring that assumptions made about the process and the decision-making that flow from them are openly debated, particularly (if conducted properly) by those people who will be affected by them. Nevertheless, the time required to carry out such an assessment is often far greater than is acceptable to politicians and fund-holders. Paradoxically, this issue is particularly relevant in the culture of target-setting that has pervaded public services for the last decade or so.

Current and future health trends in the UK were recently examined in relation to NHS resources allocation by Wanless (2004). This document was a report to the Prime Minister, Secretary of State for Health and the Chancellor of the Exchequer, and represented the first time that such a cross-departmental investigation had been commissioned. It provides a valuable insight into the state of health policy in the UK at the time of writing. Despite the title, *Securing Good Health for the Whole Population*, the report states at the outset that it is 'focused particularly on prevention' (p. 3). In contrast to previous UK governments, inequalities in health status in the UK are core to the document's message. Nevertheless, some assumptions are remarkably unchanged from those of New Labour's predecessors. Under the heading 'Who is responsible, and what support is needed?', the official view is unequivocal:

Individuals are ultimately responsible for their own and their children's health ... people need to be supported more actively to make better decisions about their own health and welfare because there are widespread, systematic failures that influence the decisions individuals currently make. (p. 4)

Moreover, these 'failures' are identified in a way that many health promoters might see as simplistic, victim-blaming and anachronistic:

These failures include a lack of full information, the difficulty individuals have in considering fully the wider social costs of particular behaviours, engrained social attitudes not conducive to individuals pursuing healthy lifestyles and addictions. (p. 4)

We believe that many readers of these statements, particularly those working in health promotion, the NHS generally, in statutory social services or in the voluntary sector, may have at least three points of issue with such a generalisation. First, consider the assertion that individuals are 'ultimately responsible' for their own health. It is likely that anyone with a disability or suffering from chronic disease, or who is living in the state of relative poverty that afflicts an alarming proportion of UK citizens, or who simply lives alone and is lonely, might support a different view, particularly if subscribing to Ewles and Simnett's concepts of health discussed earlier in this chapter. Second, consider cigarette smoking as an example: in the 21st century, do all smokers in the UK smoke because they are unaware of the dangers of smoking, and because they have never been told of the social costs of their habit? Would being told 'the full facts' immediately assure their lasting abstinence? Third, consider the notion that if people do not conform to government-approved social norms, then a 'failure' of 'widespread, systematic' proportions must have occurred. To many, such a suggestion might be disturbing in terms of the rights of individuals vis-à-vis the wishes of government. Nevertheless, Wanless makes his view of the role of government with regard to prescribing social norms clear:

Shifting social norms is a legitimate activity for Government where it has set for the nation objectives for behavioural change. (p. 4)

Apart from the obvious tautology of this statement, the idea of a government 'setting national objectives for behavioural change' may well be perceived by some as disturbing in terms of individual freedom.

Nevertheless, it would misrepresent the Wanless report to suggest that it has reverted to a stance toward the promotion of health as victim-blaming and as focused on individual behaviour, as was the case 20 years ago. The report explicitly lists the players seen as vital for the improvement of the nation's health, requiring:

wide ranging action by health and care services, government – national and local, media, business, society at large, families and the voluntary and community sector. (p. 4)

While it is not obvious who 'society at large' or the 'community sector' might be, there is in this document an explicit recognition that poverty, inequalities, as well as social and cultural factors influence health-related behaviours, rather than solely individual choice.

Moreover, the report is realistic about the limited success (to date) of public health measures, and public health medicine, in bringing about substantive changes to health status, a theme to which we will return later in this volume. It also makes clear the need for an evidence-based approach to developing public health policy and sets out responsibilities for how the NHS may tackle the major causes of premature mortality in the UK, such as coronary heart disease and certain cancers. Importantly, the report also berates the loss of the former Health Education Authority as an identifiable focus for health information. Nevertheless, the report gives little real consideration to ways of improving the quality of people's lives, *other than* by reducing the incidence of disease and disability.

Taking health promotion forward

Throughout this book, we argue the case for a different kind of health promotion activity. Of course we do not suggest that reducing the incidence of serious diseases is unimportant, nor unworthy of increased attention. On the contrary, and in common with all those concerned with improving health, we warmly welcome the current redirection of NHS and other statutory resources towards preventing, rather than simply treating, disease. But we also make the case for taking this trend one stage further. We argue for a properly funded, additional approach to health promotion programmes: those whose *primary focus* is improving the quality of people's day-to-day lives in areas which they have helped to identify, rather than solely aiming to prevent disease. We believe it is in this way that health promotion may be taken forward.

TWO Health, disease and illness: the voice of authority

Be careful about reading health books. You may die of a misprint.

Mark Twain

Thirty years ago a fair, gangly teenager sat in his doctor's waiting room, waiting to be treated for some minor ailment. On the wall were posters of those particularly gaudy Technicolor hues peculiar to the 1960s, showing various items of food – apples, carrots, cheese, fish, a loaf of bread. With reassuring confidence, the boy was advised to consume lots of cheese and milk 'for healthy bones', to eat plenty of red meat 'for protein' and to avoid too much bread or too many potatoes because these items were 'fattening'. Yet within the space of a few decades, the balance of human nutritional requirements has apparently completely reversed. Last week, in the same waiting room, the same (now grey, middle-aged) individual was presented with an only marginally less meretricious poster. With equally self-assured confidence, the viewer is advised to eat lots of bread and potatoes for 'dietary fibre', to eat less red meat because of its 'high cholesterol content' and to consume dairy products in such restricted quantities that would make all but the least hedonistic person's diet miserable.

The World Health Organization's definition of health described in Chapter 1 is useful in that it introduces both positive and negative aspects of health and disease. It also directs attention to three major dimensions of any adequate definition – the physical, mental and social, and to the distinction between health and disease. As we have seen, however, it suffers from the customary incompleteness that accompanies efforts at providing concise definitions of concepts that are notoriously difficult to delineate. Furthermore, the WHO definition reflects a particular viewpoint. It is couched in conventional medical language and is limited by the concerns of a particular epoch. Thus, disease is mentioned, but not illness per se.

Another approach to the issue of definitions is to consider the range of models that have been proposed. Various professional groups, such as biomedical researchers, sociologists, psychologists, as well as lay persons, all construct models of health, disease and illness. Within professions these may be contested according to theoretical and methodological preferences. Models held by lay persons will also vary as they reflect particular cultural and social contexts.

In the first section of this chapter our attention will focus on models employed by health professionals. We begin with a brief consideration of the rise of the medical or biomedical model, and then examine an array of social science approaches. Our aim is to identify the strands of thought that have contributed to the understanding of people working in health promotion rather than to select a single best model. In the following section we compare these models with some of those held by lay people and then consider the implications for professional/lay interactions. Following this examination we review the factors that have contributed to the medicalisation of health concerns and to governmental strategies which aim to improve the nation's health.

Distinguishing health from disease and illness

Historians debate the precise date of the establishment of scientific medicine but Porter (1995) has argued 'that medicine was implicated in the Enlightenment formulation of the positivistic human sciences' (p. 77). Sydenham, an English physician writing in the 17th century, argued that diseases, which he considered to exist as discoverable entities, could be classified in the fashion of plants or animals (Smith, 2002).

In his highly influential book, *The Birth of the Clinic*, Foucault (1973) asserted that it was the reform of the Paris Hospital in 1794 that gave a 'scientific gaze' to medicine. Despite proposing a later date and being focused upon medicine in France, there is little doubt that Foucault has documented the developing dominance of a scientific view of the body as part of nature and the abandonment of magic, mysticism and faith in dealing with bodily ills.

In the 19th century medical knowledge and practice moved away from an earlier reliance on tradition and textual authority and embraced systematic observation and experimentation. Medical empiricism became the order of the day. After Pasteur's innovations in bacteriology, illness was transformed and specimens of disease took centre stage. By the middle of the 19th century pathology and disease, rather than sick people, were the objects of medical attention. The ill person had become a challenge to be diagnosed or categorised. Since the body could be defined as diseased, the negative of healthy, it was described as pathological or abnormal. Implicit in this disease model is a notion of a population against which the pathological can be identified. We have already noted a positive dimension as health, but the concept of normality implies a further aspect, one that considers health in terms of populations, distributions and norms.

The focus of the biomedical model is disease, identified as pathology; by and large the subjective experience of illness is ignored. Thus a person with an undiagnosed medically defined disease, such as prostate cancer, might feel healthy and only become anxious and indeed feel ill upon receiving the results of a screening test indicative of disease. On the other hand, sufferers often seek a scientific diagnosis of an identifiable disease to legitimise their symptoms (Aronowitz, 1998). A disease label may turn blame into sympathy and provide a legitimate explanation for failure to meet obligations, be they domestic or occupational (Smith, 2002).

Subjectively experienced illnesses such as Myalgic Encephalomyelitis (ME) or Chronic Fatigue Syndrome (CFS) have posed a challenge to the diagnostic process of scientific medicine. The reality of the subjective experience has been questioned and CFS has not yet gained complete acceptance in the medical world (Smith, 2002). Although individuals had reported feeling ill, and experienced great discomfort, until recently medical scientists had failed to identify a specific disease. We return to the distinction between disease and illness in relation to social science models and to the subjective aspect of health and illness when we consider lay persons' definitions in the next section of this chapter.

The disease focus of the medical model is illustrated by the definition proffered by a junior doctor when asked to describe a healthy person. He replied, 'Someone who has not been completely worked up' (Kolata, 2001: 2). Taken to extremes, the medical or biomedical model leads to other strange conclusions. Prior (2000) has argued that contemporary practices surrounding health, disease and death can be read as an assertion that death is conquerable. He reaches this conclusion by first noting that, officially, no one dies of 'old age'; it is not a disease. The administrative requirements surrounding the completion of a death certificate demand that death be attributed to a specific set of diseases. The International Classification of Disease, now in a tenth revision (ICD-10), is the system used in England and Wales, in the United States, and many other nations. Just as individuals are held to be responsible for risks relating to personal health, illness, and disease, so too with the risk of death. In contemporary society death has been demoted. As medical science comes to 'conquer' disease, the illusion is created that individuals may control death through the avoidance of risky behaviour that leads to disease and hence death. Although this brief summary may lose some of the force of Prior's carefully argued presentation, the seductive power of the medical model of disease can easily be discerned.

The widespread use of ICD-10 may create the impression that the identification of disease is straightforward, but the medical profession acknowledges that the boundary between disease and non-disease is difficult to identify. In a special issue of the *British Medical Journal* that boundary was explored and 'the slipperiness of the notion of disease' was shown (Smith, 2002: 883). In an earlier *BMJ* survey of lay and professional people, few of 38 terms were identified unequivocally as diseases (Campbell, Scadding & Roberts, 1979). Positive identifications were given for tuberculosis and malaria, but fewer than 20% of people completing the survey thought that lead poisoning, skull fracture or blindness were diseases. As we noted above, when we discussed CFS, sufferers may gain benefits from a disease label but there are also liabilities in terms of employment, financial arrangements such as insurance and borrowing, and the individual sense of being damaged. Thus the contemporary disposition to classify people's suffering and problems as disease may have both negative and positive implications. We will return to this issue when we consider the medicalisation of health.

In the second half of the 20th century anthropologists, sociologists and psychologists all staked claims to health issues. By the end of the century the emphasis within sociology had shifted away from the group or population to individuals and their responsibilities for ensuring their health and avoiding risks (Prior, 2000). Busfield (2000) describes four explanatory schema within medical sociology:

- individual health-behaviour
- individual-level attributes and circumstances
- material environment and resource distribution
- social relations and subjectivity.

She laments the emphasis on individual health-behaviour, which has had limited success, and emphasises the importance of resources and social relations. Medical sociologists have come to describe their domain as the sociology of health and illness while a new professional division within the British Psychological Society bears the title Health Psychology.

Atkinson (1995) offers an insight into the distinction between disease and illness in his description of the formation of their object of study by medical sociologists. He describes the process in terms of a set of binary oppositions. He identified these as 'disease/illness; biology/culture; signs/ symptoms; professional/lay; medical/sociological' (p. 23). Social scientists claimed culture as their own, along with illness, symptoms, and lay persons. The boundary between medicine and the social sciences was clarified when the medical model became the biomedical model. Thus identified, the vast enterprise of medical research and practice was distinguished from health concerns within the domains of anthropologists, sociologists, and psychologists.

Although this strategy was successful in establishing the identity of medical sociology in the 1960s, Atkinson has argued that it was restricting. The view that disease belonged to medicine as it was part of the natural world, while illness was viewed as a cultural construction, failed to recognise that disease too had been created through the social interaction of medical discourse and practice.

Further attention was drawn to the social dimensions of medicine in the 1970s as part of the surge of criticisms against biomedicine and the assumptions that were inherent in medical practice (Illich, 1976). Although the scientific basis of medical research was rarely challenged directly, the practice of medicine came under increasing scrutiny. In a now classic text, McKeown (1976) questioned the effectiveness of medical practice and offered evidence that it was hygiene, nutrition and controlled reproduction that had been the most potent factors in reducing mortality (death rates) in Western societies in the 20th century.

Illich (1976) offered a stronger critique that included both the natural and the social worlds. In its time Illich's attack gained wide acceptance and led to many later developments. The term medicalisation came into use as Illich described the power of medical research and practice. Arguing from both a medical and a Marxist perspective, he not only pointed out that powerful modern drugs can have serious side effects, but he also noted that the hierarchical structure of medicine encouraged passivity and acceptance of established medical practice among patients. Individuals failed to challenge 'scientific' opinion. Illich's critique, and various other theoretical strands within sociology, including the phenomenological approach of Berger and Luckman (1967), have contributed to the current dominance of a social constructionist model of health and illness.

Nettleton (1995) has suggested that social constructionism has taken the sociology of health and illness a long way. The positivist epistemology of the biomedical model was seen as part of modernism. The challenge to a single valid truth about disease and to a history of medical knowledge that reflects a continuous progress towards such truth is at the core of the social constructionist project. Alongside it runs the belief that social relations are mediated by medical knowledge and that social relations influence biomedical research and practice.

Beyond social constructionism, the very certainties of health and illness may dissolve in the postmodernist perspective. This quotation from Fox (1998) illustrates the challenge of postmodernism:

> I shall speak not of a health fabricated by the body-with-organs, but of *arche-health*, an unfolding which is more than 'health', which

cannot be spoken because to speak it would inscribe it, and of *nomads,* subjectivities resisting and refusing discourse not patients but impatients. (p. 9, emphasis in original)

Before we rush to discount such an arcane view of health and illness and accept social constructionism, it is worth noting that there have been critics of this important model within medical sociology. Atkinson has argued for a more complex model that recognises both the material reality upon which scientific knowledge is predicated as well as the social forces that guide its formulation. To illustrate this contention he has cited research which showed that the attribution of disease labels is determined not by nature but through negotiation. For example, he highlighted Hunt's (1985) study of the diagnosis of hypoglycemia, and her view that disease labels are cognitive constructs which vary among physicians themselves.

Health psychology generally provides a more empirical and quantitative account of health, disease and illness than the often epistemologically sophisticated and demanding discussions of medical sociologists. In her text on health psychology, Ogden (1996) posed the question: 'What does it mean to be healthy?' In constructing a reply she drew upon a study in which healthy young adults were asked their definitions (Lau, 1995). It yielded evidence to support Ogden's assertion that for most people in the Western world being healthy is the norm and that beliefs about illness are framed within the context of health. We will pursue the content of lay persons' beliefs about health and disease in the section that follows. For the moment, Ogden's approach serves as evidence of the positivist nature of the health psychologists' approach to the study of health and disease. The empirical and quantitative approach of much of health psychology implicitly shares the rationalist, scientific epistemology of the biomedical model.

In a carefully reasoned textbook on health promotion it is argued that the pursuit of health, defined as positive subjective well-being, cannot be its ultimate professional goal (Downie, Tannahill & Tannahill, 1996). To accept such a conclusion would imply that success lay in the mass administration of heroin to the population. In countering such a notion of 'narcotic-induced euphoria' (p. 18) the authors argue that *true* well-being involves and reflects a quality which they describe as empowerment and that it has social and political dimensions. Empowerment involves having control over one's life, being able to exercise choice in terms of what one does and is, and allows scope for development. It usually involves having friends, a degree of physical comfort and freedom from arbitrary governmental decisions. Their formulation provides a preview of themes to be developed in later chapters.

Lay and professional definitions of disease and illness

Blaxter's (1995a) study described in Chapter 1 is a useful starting point in the comparison of ordinary people's definitions of disease and illness with those of health professionals. The individuals participating in her representative sample were asked questions about a person they could identify as healthy and then about their own health. Once again the dichotomy between the scientific-positivistic and the subjective-individual appears. Blaxter reminds the reader of a fundamental difference between the biomedical model of health and 'the looser more holistic model' held by lay people. An example of the difference is provided by one of her respondents who described themselves as healthy despite having a clinically recognised disease – diabetes.

The distinction Blaxter has drawn between the two models of illness, the biomedical and the holistic model, reflects two ideal types that have a history within medicine. In a revealing account of the changing meaning of specific diseases, Aronowitz (1998) contends that patients and doctors negotiate between the two models. He labels the first 'illness as a specific disease', and the second, 'individual sickness'. Among historians of medicine the first is described as ontological, indicating the specific nature of particular diseases, a concern with the thing, in itself. The disease exists as a platonic ideal. The second is also idealised and labelled the physiological or holistic model. It concerns individuals' adaptation to their environment and recognises individual idiosyncrasy. The respondent who reported being both diabetic and healthy demonstrated that the two function side by side, just as Aronowitz contends. Aronowitz, who is medically qualified, stresses the dialectical relationship between the two models in the social and scientific construction of disease.

Lay beliefs about health and illness are frequently contrasted with biomedical knowledge. Early studies of beliefs undertaken by medical sociologists drew upon the use of the term in anthropological studies of culturally diverse belief systems. Good (1994) has argued that the concept of belief was largely untheorised in these early studies and that anthropologists had often used the concept 'belief', in opposition to scientific knowledge. However, research has revealed that lay people, when considering health and illness, employ both folk beliefs and their understanding of medical knowledge.

An early and influential study of lay beliefs of health and illness was undertaken by Herzlich (1973) in France. The social psychological concept of social representations that Moscovici had developed from Durkheim's theory of collective representations provided the theoretical framework of the study. Herzlich's research was particularly significant in the 1970s as she had not selected a patient group as the object of her attention and she had sought beliefs about health as well as about illness, which had been the focus of most research at that time.

Herzlich (1973: 63) described three representations of health that she identified from interviews with 80 middle-class people living primarily in Paris. She labelled these:

- health-in-a-vacuum
- reserve of health
- equilibrium.

The first was associated with being, the second with having and the third with doing. The already familiar definition of health as the absence of illness was described as 'health-in-a-vacuum'. The social representation of health as 'reserve of health' included biological endowment but also strength and vitality. 'Equilibrium' concerns physical well-being, good humour, activity and good social relations. Clearly Herzlich's findings foreshadow dimensions identified in health definitions which were later described by Blaxter, including reserve, fitness, vitality and social relationships.

There is no doubt that Herzlich's study of health beliefs has been influential both in terms of method and content, but additional factors have shaped the current emphasis on health beliefs among researchers. Bury (1997) has suggested that the factors leading to a shift in research interest from lay beliefs about illness to those concerning health included the development of health promotion, the problems associated with the provision of health care, and issues within medical practice itself.

Before moving on to the next section we return to Smith's report of the *BMJ* study of 'non-diseases' (2002). This research reflects a concern with the labelling of individuals' problems as disease entities among medical practitioners. It was also undertaken to demonstrate the difficulty in defining disease. Perhaps one of the most interesting results was the finding that some conditions that already appear in recognised disease classifications were among the 200 non-diseases suggested by editors and readers of the *BMJ*. Health, disease and illness are concepts that both lay people and health professionals struggle to define. They are influenced by social and cultural factors as well as by the growing body of biomedical knowledge and practice, and they change over time.

But the last word on definitions of illness and disease is yet to be written (Macleod et al., 2002). Researchers followed the health of 5600 middle-aged men over a 20-year period. Initially self-reports were used to assess the men's levels of stress and their accounts of symptoms of illness. Initial results supported the medical belief that there is a link between stress and disease. Men reporting more stress reported more symptoms. The surprise came when medical records were examined 20 years later. Rates of heart disease and deaths from heart disease were actually lower among those men who had reported higher stress levels and more symptoms. A puzzling outcome and one that on first examination questions the validity of self-reports. An important question remains. Did the men's heightened awareness of stress and symptoms result in health care behaviours that improved their outcomes?

Implications for the therapeutic relationship

Changes in society, including the influence of lay and professional beliefs about health, illness and disease, have shaped social science research into the therapeutic relationship. When the topic was first examined in the middle of the 20th century, patients as well as nurses and other health-professionals accepted a hierarchical structure that placed medical doctors at its apex. Generally, social life in the 1950s and early 1960s was more deferential than it is now. Doctors and nurses might address patients by their first names but titles were used in response. Today patients are ready to question professionals with information gained from support groups or from the internet, and to challenge outcomes with recourse to law.

Models of the patient/doctor relationship employed in social science research reflect the dominance of different theoretical and methodological approaches within the sociology of medicine. Until the middle of the 20th century sociologists and psychologists had shown limited interest in issues of health. It was the American sociologist Talcott Parsons (1951) who first gave medicine a prominent position in his structural-functional model of society. Parsons construed illness as a kind of abnormality or deviance and described the function of medicine as curing the disturbance and returning the sick to health so that they could fulfil their roles in society. The sick role was identified as entailing two rights and two obligations (Hardey, 1998). The rights were defined as, firstly, exemption from expectations that they would fulfil their normal roles, such as work, and, secondly, that they would not be blamed for their illness and that they could expect help in regaining health. The right to be exempt from blame may lie behind support group efforts to reach medical consensus on the nature of conditions such as Chronic Fatigue Syndrome. The obligations of patients were to seek appropriate attention from a doctor and co-operate with the prescribed course of treatment and recover as quickly as possible. Social values of a collective orientation, universalism and affective neutrality were held to ensure the successful operation of such a system.

The ideals presented in the Parsonian model are rarely met and conflicting voices can readily be heard. In the next chapter we examine evidence that health and illness are influenced by position in society. Government rhetoric has often been more individualistic. In the 1992 government document *Health of the Nation*, individuals were exhorted to help themselves avoid the sick role. A celebrated departure from the idealised values of the structural-functional model was the suggestion that smokers, who were viewed as bringing illness upon themselves, be denied heart bypass surgery (Underwood & Bailey, 1993).

Long before the question of treatment for smokers was raised, social scientists challenged the ideals of structural-functional analysis. Freidson (1970) proposed that it was suppressed conflict, rather than consensus, that characterised the therapeutic relationship. He focused upon the different worlds which doctors and patients inhabited. He described the lay concern with illness and contrasted this with the medical world of disease. Attention to the differing worlds of lay and professional people also brought into focus the different social and cultural worlds inhabited by lay people.

The conflict model drew attention to the problems experienced by practitioners as well as those encountered by patients. Bloor and Horobin (1975) reported that GPs considered that they were called upon excessively to make night visits and that they experienced considerable frustration as well as conflict in their interaction with patients. An important source of frustration lay in the wish of GPs that their patients present with a clear idea of their problem and not 'waste' the time of their doctor with frivolous complaints. A quarter of a century later this concern has been quantified in a study demonstrating the patient complaint categories that GPs query as legitimate descriptions of disease (Smith, 2002). Such conflicts challenge the Parsonian consensus model even when professional manner or patient deference may temporarily resolve them.

Conflict models derived from Marxist and feminist perspectives also came to the fore in the 1970s. Bury (1997) has described research in hospital medicine in which Waitzkin characterised the therapeutic relationship 'as a means of reinforcing dominant ideologies rather than helping to reinforce shared values' (1979: 90). In this discourse the rational, scientific biomedical model of disease is viewed as dominant but as occupying a restricted position in society. Thus Waitzkin asserted that medicine silenced protest by de-politicing social relationships. This may be a valid criticism but adopting such a wider perspective, one involving interpersonal and social factors, risks the accusation of the medicalisation of everyday life. This issue is explored in the next section.

Feminists (e.g., Oakley, 1980) took issue with the control of women's bodies that male doctors exercised through the medicalisation of pregnancy and childbirth. Once again it was conflict rather than consensus that was held to characterise the therapeutic relationship. Radical feminists attributed male control of women's bodies to patriarchal values. Some feminists even challenged reformist campaigns for the treatment of women by women practitioners, arguing that medical education imparted similar values to men and women alike. Analysis of the therapeutic relationship, informed by critical theory (Habermas, 1970), examined the consequences of its fundamental inequality. Ideological distortion of seemingly objective medical communication was held to be a consequence of hierarchy.

Both the consensual model proposed by Parsons and the conflict model first expounded by Freidson construe the patient as passive or at least deferential when confronted by the superior knowledge of medical practitioners. This is exacerbated further in the structure of the National Health Service where the gatekeeping role of GPs determines access to hospital medicine. A challenge to both of these views of the therapeutic relationship comes from the interpretative or micro-level analysis of patient/doctor relationships. Despite conflict being an element and patients having to negotiate with professionals to gain a referral or other outcome, they also often report satisfaction with the encounter. As Bury describes it, 'Negotiation implies both the presence of conflict and the willingness to work towards an agreement, if not in establishing a consensus' (1997: 98).

This largely historical discussion has been grounded in the doctor/patient relationship and has not considered three major influences that may change the therapeutic relationship significantly in the future. Bury (1997) identifies these as:

- the demographics of ageing populations and increasing chronic illness
- availability of medical knowledge and alternative therapies
- evaluation of medical practice and accountability.

Chronic illness places responsibility for management more squarely with the patient. Any confidence thus gained may well change patients' perceptions of the importance of their doctors. Allied to such change is the availability of both scientific and medical knowledge and other treatments. Karpf (1988) has reported that doctors themselves have become much more willing to dispense medical knowledge via the mass media. Allied to the public availability of information is the scientific evaluation of medical practice. Treatment may become a more contractual arrangement with doctors offering patients specific information about risks and outcomes.

The medicalisation of health

The vignette at the beginning of this chapter, set in a GP's surgery, brings to life the voice of medical authority. It illustrates one of the main tenets of the medicalisation thesis, that medical jurisdiction has broadened over the two centuries of scientific biomedicine and that spheres of life such as sexuality, alcoholism and old age, to say nothing of diet, now fall within its domain. Williams and Calnan (1996) have speculated that the search for genetic precursors of disease and disability will only extend medical jurisdiction further.

As we have already noted, in the 1970s Illich (1976) described modern medicine as a calculated effort to defeat death, disease and suffering. He argued that before the rise of modern medicine all societies had developed means of dealing with these events, but that in modern industrial societies ways of coping had been handed over to the medical establishment. In seeking to explain medicalisation, Illich looked beyond the medical profession to wider trends in society, to industrialisation and bureaucratisation. As we have already noted, other efforts to explain medicalisation have followed Foucault and focused on issues of social control, be they from a Marxist or feminist perspective.

Now, more than a quarter of a century later, the agenda of health promotion activity could be viewed as yet another manifestation of establishment control, of medicalisation. Before accepting such a conclusion we review an analysis of the contemporary relationship between biomedicine and the lay public (Williams & Calnan, 1996). These authors draw upon Giddens' (1990; 1991) theory of 'late' modernity and Beck's (1992) theory of risk to question whether lay people are passively dependent believers in the voice of authority.

Williams and Calnan argue that the strength of Giddens' analysis comes from his rejection of postmodernism and from his creative theorising of 'late' modernity. The hallmark of this late or high modernity is social reflexivity – 'the susceptibility of most aspects of social activity, and material relations with nature, to chronic revision in the light of new information and knowledge' (Williams & Calnan, 1996: 1612). The subjective self and self-identity are also foci of Giddens' analysis. It is this combination of Giddens' concerns with the self, knowledge and society that provide the foundation for Williams and Calnan's critique of the medicalisation thesis. The emphasis on reflexivity implies that beliefs and practices are subject to continual scrutiny and revision, as illustrated in the vignette at the beginning of this chapter. The attitude of reflexivity leads to radical doubt. The certainties of custom and tradition are not replaced. Given an attitude of radical doubt, issues of trust and risk take on added significance. In such a world lay beliefs about medicine become more open and complex as trust and doubt result in both hope and despair.

Beck's theory (1992) is used to explore the concept of risk (Williams & Calnan, 1996). As we have already noted, Illich described all societies as dealing with death, disease and suffering. What has changed is beliefs about these risks and the nature of risk. In the past, calamities could be blamed on nature, the Gods or fate. Today we seek explanations in terms of man-made risks such as climate change or pollution. Modernity is marked, Beck holds, not only by risks that we create but by a concerted effort through specific calculation and governmental intervention to regulate them. Modern medicine, with its powerful pharmacopoeia, offers the benefits and risks that Beck has described. Modern drugs list, alongside ingredients and instruction for use, all the known side-effects that have been reported.

Health promotion is no more free of suspicion than is the medical profession. Smoking cessation advice to pregnant women is met with complex lay beliefs, including the desire for a small baby, alongside anecdotal evidence of smokers who produce normal babies (Lucas, 1994). The processes of doubt, re-valuation and risk assessment characterise modern society wherever the voice of authority originates.

The media, as purveyors of knowledge, play an increasingly important role in mediating lay experience. A positive consequence of the increased media participation in medical issues is the 're-skilling' of lay populations. One result of the widespread use of the internet is patient awareness of new medical procedures and drugs almost as soon as they are introduced. In the information society health promotion can function to re-empower individuals and provide them with knowledge that could help them reduce the risk of illness and improve their health. In the discussion that follows we will consider some of the influences that shape public health concerns.

Before relegating the concept of medicalisation to the 20th century we examine one further challenge to it. Moynihan, Heath and Henry (2002), in their analysis of the role of the pharmaceutical industry in shaping health care, introduce the term 'disease mongering'. They argue that in order to increase corporate profitability drug companies:

- turn ordinary ailments into medical problems
- see mild symptoms as being more serious
- treat personal problems as medical matters
- describe risks as diseases
- use occurrence statistics to maximise their markets.

From admittedly anecdotal evidence, they argue for disease mongering to be employed to describe such corporate activity, rather than medicalisation. These authors claim that global pharmaceutical companies are active in the definition of new diseases, fund studies of drug effectiveness, support leading researchers as well as patient groups and specific disease foundations, and both advertise and provide prizes to journalists who produce media accounts of these diseases. The media play an important role in forming lay beliefs, but medical professionals as well as patient groups are targeted by the media too and directly influenced by pharmaceutical companies.

Osteoporosis, or reduced bone mass, is only one of Moynihan, Heath and Henry's examples of disease mongering. They draw upon a press release from Osteoporosis Australia, a medical foundation supported by pharmaceutical companies, to illustrate their argument. The press release described osteoporosis as 'a silent thief' which could sneak up on a person and destroy their quality of life and health (Moynihan, Heath & Henry, 2002: 889). The 10-question checklist that accompanied the article included the question: are you a menopausal woman? A positive response to this item alone was followed by the suggestion that a visit to a doctor and screening for osteoporosis was indicated.

The definition of osteoporosis provided by the World Health Organization states that disease is present if a person's bone mineral density measurement is 1.6 standard deviations below the mean for normal young adult white women. The diagnostic use of this criterion means that large numbers of menopausal women are defined as osteoporotic. It is worth noting that the WHO committee that produced the criteria for disease presence was funded in part by three pharmaceutical companies. Doctors are thus likely to prescribe a variety of chemical solutions despite limited research evidence of their effectiveness. One four-year study based upon the drug alendronate found an absolute reduction of only 1.7% in the incidence of radiographic vertebral fractures. It is the controversy surrounding diagnosis, the limited evidence of therapeutic efficacy, and the profits drug companies accrue, that have led Moynihan and his colleagues to attack the strategy of global pharmaceutical corporations as disease mongering rather than medicalisation.

Were we to accept Williams and Calnan's (1996) argument that lay people are no longer 'simply passive or active, dependent or independent, believers or sceptics, rather they are a complex mixture of all these things (and much more besides)' (p. 1619), we might relegate medicalisation to the dustbin of history. However, the report of Moynihan, Heath and Henry (2002) is a warning that even active, independent and sceptical lay and professional persons alike may be taken in by clever promotions and that the hunt for disease is not yet over. But their paper also reported that calcium and vitamin D supplements, smoking cessation and weight-bearing exercise are known to have therapeutic effects. Would health promotion efforts to increase lay awareness of these therapeutic agencies be construed as medicalisation? Has the concept had its day in a questioning society poised between the desire for health and the fear of illness?

Public health 'medicine' and medical education

Holland (2002) provides a detailed historical comparison of public health training and research in the UK and in the USA. He notes that the development of public health research capacity has differed markedly between the two countries. Immediately following the First World War, there were 16 universities in the UK containing medical schools. Outside London, almost all of these had academic departments concerned with epidemiology and/or public health, and those in Newcastle, Liverpool, Leeds, Sheffield and Bristol had joint appointments with the health department of the local city. In these cases, the departmental professor was also the local Medical Officer of Health. Clearly, at that time the prevalence of infectious diseases was reflected in the nature of public health appointments and thus in London, particularly, there were joint posts with bacteriology and immunology departments. It is noteworthy that in 1928, the London School of Tropical Medicine changed its title to the London School of Hygiene and Tropical Medicine. In the years that followed, the School expanded, primarily in bacteriology.

Following the Second World War, an expansion occurred in public health teaching in most British universities, but the emphasis on infectious and industrial diseases remained. A number of universities adopted the title 'Social Medicine' for this discipline, including Oxford, Birmingham and Dublin; this term was expanded to 'Social and Industrial Medicine' at (perhaps predictably) Sheffield, and even 'Social and Preventive Medicine' at Belfast.

The size and staffing of medical school public health departments has expanded greatly since the 1970s. Clarke and Kurinczuk (1992) found that by the beginning of the 1990s there were 121 medically-qualified academics, 36 statisticians, 23 social scientists and 36 other staff employed in this field. However, while this is generally seen by public health physicians as evidence of a greater appreciation of their skills, expertise and potential contribution to the nation's health, we would argue that by the end of the 20th century such a perspective had become less appropriate than it was at the beginning of it. Few people in the developed world, and certainly in the UK, now die from infectious or industrial diseases. We would argue that of the 180 identifiably professional staff in this survey, *only* 23 (13%) have a specific background in the social sciences. By contrast, 121 (67%) of these appointments were held by medical practitioners. Throughout this volume we have emphasised the key role of social, psychological and societal factors in determining most people's health status in the UK today. From this viewpoint, it could be argued that at the time of Clark and Kurinczuk's study, over two-thirds of these appointments were held by individuals for whom a substantial majority of their (highly expensive and publicly-funded) training was largely irrelevant to the areas of expertise they are required to possess. Holland (2002: 19), perhaps unconsciously, concurs with this observation by noting that 'the nomenclature of the subject [public health teaching] has changed many times over the past 100 years, even if the content remains the same'.

This point has been made, in a much more inflammatory manner, by the well-known health economist Alan Maynard. In a journal read very widely by British health service senior managers, Maynard (1999) questioned whether the NHS can afford public health medicine as it is organised currently. He suggested that the existing system poses a double burden to the NHS in that not only are medical doctors less appropriately qualified to perform current public health functions than are, for example, graduates in sociology, statistics, management and economics, but that they also cost twice as much to employ and far more still to train. Maynard went on to describe public health medicine as what he calls an excessively well-paid 'medical club' inhabited by what he calls 'drains doctors'. Moreover, Maynard suggests, somewhat caustically, that, given the current shortage of GPs, the NHS would benefit greatly 'if drains folk – after suitable retraining – could be used to provide primary care in the deprived areas with which they are, apparently, so concerned' (p. 18).

Maynard concludes that:

> surely it is time to develop and use openly the [social science and economics] knowledge base rather than politely avoid a very pertinent policy issue because some feel it impolite to challenge the medical mafia. (p. 18)

The backlash to Maynard's article was perhaps predictable and was certainly vehement. Each in their turn, Hadden (1999) questioned Maynard's economic analysis, Griffiths (1999) argued that his view of public health medicine was 'sadly dated', while Eskin (1999) reminded him of the benefits brought to society by effective sewage disposal and clean drinking water (although, in our view, these developments may arguably be equally attributable to Victorian engineering as to medicine). If Maynard's tirade may have been intended to be controversial, it certainly appeared to touch a nerve: considerable debate followed in many public health departments concerning the appropriateness and equity of their structure. Moreover, Maynard was not alone in this apparent heresy.

Ainsworth (1999) is even more explicit about the limitations of a medically-dominated model of public health. It is arguable that communicable diseases represent the only part of public health work that truly requires a medical training: this is evidenced by one London health authority's recent opening up of all new public health posts (with the exception of communicable diseases) to non-medically qualified applicants. In an equally widely-read article which echoes Maynard's view, Ainsworth again reminds us that few people in the UK today die from infectious diseases. Equally caustically, he thus suggests that:

> ... without a sudden outbreak of bubonic plague, public health doctors now have very little to do. The Broad Street pump could only be discovered once. For a brief period when it looked as though AIDS would take on the proportions of a biblical plague, there was a possibility that public health might experience a renaissance, but that has proved a false dawn. (1999: 14)

Ainsworth goes on to suggest that the major causes of mortality today are diseases of old age, and that no public health measures can prevent old age. In less invidious language, however, Ainsworth poses a more serious challenge to the public health status quo:

> Public health won its great victories many decades ago, and now trades on past glory. Its remaining functions – commissioning health education, collecting health statistics and reporting on them – could be carried out just as effectively by part-time honorary public health directors. (1999: 15)

A further point made by Ainsworth juxtaposes his views of the inappropriateness of medically-driven public health departments with a question concerning the usefulness of the annual reports produced by directors of public health. These reports are statutorily-required documents, the production of which year on year provides the focus of much activity in most public health departments. He asks:

> And wouldn't it be marvellous if we could find a public health director brave enough to issue an annual report printed on just one side of A4 which said simply 'Absolutely nothing has changed since last year, and of those problems that do exist there is very little of significant value which you or I can do about them' ... More important, given the shortage of 'real' doctors, at what point will the government decide that medical practitioners currently leading unproductive and unfulfilling lives in public health would be better employed treating real patients rather than having their undoubted talents going to waste at such great public expense? (1999: 23)

While it is true that Ainsworth, like Maynard, is (perhaps deliberately) vitriolic in his criticism of public health doctors, it is anecdotally commonplace for the views so bluntly voiced by Maynard and Ainsworth to manifest as local tensions between public health doctors and clinical colleagues on an everyday basis. Moreover, their arguments do, in our view, at least bear serious consideration. They have at least increased debate and may have even contributed to the beginnings of change.

In the UK, public health has rarely been considered as the most prestigious of specialities open to medical graduates, particularly when compared to, for example, surgery or cardiology. Holland (2002: 23) draws a clear contrast to the British situation with that in the United States, both historically and in the present day: 'In contrast to the UK, physicians active in public health were often considered the elite of their profession'.

Holland goes on to list important examples, including Stephen Smith, one of the founders of the American Public Health Association, and William Welch, the Dean of Johns Hopkins School of Medicine. In the period between the wars, public health medicine was far better funded in the USA than in the UK, including considerable support from the Rockefeller Foundation.

Yet it is not only in terms of prestige and funding that public health research and practice has been more forward-looking in the USA. As long ago as 1936, the proportion of medically-qualified students in public health at Johns Hopkins was lower (63%) than that of their British counterparts in the 1990s, while the proportion of students with a medical background at the Michigan School of Public Health in 1936 was only 25% (Ludmerer, 1999). By 1919, courses in public health for non-medical professionals such as engineers were already developed in the American universities of Harvard, Yale, Michigan, Columbia and Pennsylvania (Fee & Acheson, 1991). In the USA between the late 1950s and the mid-1970s, the number of students in public health schools quadrupled, and alongside this expansion the range of work taken within the purview of public health widened to include health administration and family planning.

This latter observation is in itself an interesting commentary on differences between American and British doctors' perceptions of public health at the time and warrants a brief discussion at this point. In the UK, the state provision of contraceptive advice and services by doctors has a long and half-hearted history. The first 'birth control clinic' in London was founded by Marie Stopes in 1921. Dr Stopes was not a medical graduate, but a palaeobotanist: despite not being medically qualified, her vision overtook the disinterest of contemporary medics and she became the leading pioneer of sexual health in Britain. From these beginnings, five separate 'birth control societies' provided open clinics which later combined to form the Family Planning Association. Their aims were the improvement of maternal and child health, and the increase of marital happiness. The latter is an issue addressed only recently in mainstream sexual health promotion when compared to the treatment and prevention of disease.

In 1930, the then Ministry of Health issued a circular to local health authorities permitting them to provide contraceptive advice to women 'for whom a further pregnancy would be detrimental to health'. Despite radical changes in public attitudes towards sexuality, and the advent of oral contraceptives in the 1960s, assent was only given in 1974 to the NHS Reorganisation Bill by which family planning finally became part of the NHS. This date was three years after the Family Planning Association (a registered charity staffed largely by volunteers) had celebrated 50 years of providing sexual health services across the UK. Even sterilization, a procedure clearly the exclusive province of doctors, was only recommended for NHS provision by a working party of the Royal College of Obstetricians and Gynaecologists in 1972. At the same time, general practitioners strongly resisted suggestions that they should provide contraception on the grounds that it demeaned their status to that of barbers and sellers of rubber goods. However, such professional concerns suddenly evaporated when the government agreed to pay GPs a set fee for providing such services.

British doctors' historical selectivity in the involvement with such important public health issues, despite a concurrent insistence on their own dominance of the discipline as a whole, has been far less a feature of developing public health capacity in the USA. It is perhaps unsurprising, therefore, to note Holland's (2002) observation that, by 1988, the proportion of medical graduates in American public health schools varied from 5% at the University of Massachusetts to 46% at Harvard, with an average of only 22% across all schools. Even at this time, 8% of students in US public health schools had a nursing background, while public health nursing (as opposed to community nursing or health visiting) is still a relatively recent concept in the UK.

The American approach to education in public health reflects a much longer history of an understanding of the need for a truly (as opposed to a lip-service) multidisciplinary approach to public health and health promotion. Recognition of the limitations of a purely medical background is evidenced in Holland's (2002: 27) view:

> The acceptance that public health knowledge and its application are multidisciplinary [has] been dominant in the USA since the beginning of the twentieth century. … so that by the end of the twentieth century the great majority of both staff and students were not medically qualified.

While the situation is changing slowly in the UK, public health is still dominated by medicine. Non-medically qualified Directors of Public Health are still rare, and as Maynard so pointedly observes, non-medically qualified staff working in public health have lower status and are generally paid far less than their medical colleagues for doing very similar tasks, for which the latter are often less appropriately prepared.

Perhaps more importantly, a shift from solely preventing disease towards improving health and well-being remains less likely to occur. It is only by facing and dealing with such anomalies honestly that major changes can be made to the effectiveness of health promotion programmes in the UK.

THREE   Health, social indicators and the quality of life

Again and again I have found that 'statistically significant' truth (often with the exceptions – the 'outliers' – excluded from the calculation for statistical reasons) had little relevance to the truth of my unique encounter with the person of flesh and blood before me.

Irvin D Yalom

In Glasgow, a 60-year-old woman (we'll call her Margaret) attended a clinic once a week to receive treatment for a minor ailment. She was sprightly in manner, well-dressed and always cheerful, despite a constant struggle to make ends meet financially.

Over a period of two months, the clinic staff noticed that Margaret seemed to be using more and more of a particularly pungent perfume. One day, the scent became so overpowering that during her treatment, we very cautiously enquired what brand of perfume it was. Margaret began to cry, and asked 'Can I show you something?' She opened her blouse, and removed several layers of stained bandages and padding from her breast. Finally, she revealed what was obviously a large, fungating tumour. The lesion appeared advanced and had a purulent, offensive discharge.

Margaret explained that she had been widowed 15 years ago, and since then had lived alone. She had one daughter, who was a lone parent with two small children. Margaret earned a living stacking shelves in a local supermarket, and the flexibility of her working hours enabled her to collect her grandchildren from school each day, so that her daughter could work. She had not sought treatment for her tumour partly because she was afraid of being given a diagnosis of cancer, but primarily because subsequent hospitalisation would have prevented her from looking after her grandchildren, thereby compromising her daughter's employment and much-needed income. We encouraged Margaret to seek treatment immediately, but Margaret died a few months later.

The aim of health promotion interventions is to help people improve their health. However, the outcome measures that are generally used to determine the effectiveness of interventions usually assess the incidence of death and disease, that is to say mortality and morbidity rates. The specific aims of such interventions are to reduce the rate of death from disease, particularly coronary heart disease (CHD) and cancer, or to change behaviours that carry high risks to health such as cigarette smoking and being overweight or obese. As we will observe in discussing the work of Marmot and Wilkinson (1999) on the effects of social class on health, the behaviour that has been measured contributes little to improving health or longevity. What has been missing from efforts to effect change through health promotion are measures of the quality of people's lives and their perceived states of health. As we already noted in Chapter 2, the biomedical model focuses instead on the diagnosis of disease rather than on measuring health.

Mortality/Morbidity

The terms that epidemiologists use to describe rates of death and disease are mortality and morbidity. Deaths, as well as births and marriages, have been recorded for a long time. In the UK the law has required registration of births and deaths since 1874. Although death statistics were gathered in parts of the USA from the beginning of the 20th century, complete coverage of the country was only achieved in 1933.

Epidemiology, or population medicine, depends upon the classification of disease. In Chapter 2 we noted that the criteria of the *International Classification of Diseases and Related Health Problems (ICD)* are used to assign causes of death, both immediate and underlying, to disease categories for death certificates in England and Wales. The international acceptance of this system allows group comparisons by age, gender, social class, ethnicity, race, occupation, etc., within societies as well as cross-nationally. A more detailed system has been developed in the US that is completely compatible with *ICD9*. Its full title is *International Classification of Diseases, 9th Revision, Clinical Modification. ICD9.CM* provides additional clinical information needed for epidemiological research into morbidity statistics for medical librarians and for care-funding bodies.

Morbidity rates, or disease statistics, are dependent upon reports of health service activity. Physicians are legally required to notify the occurrence of only a relatively few infectious diseases. There has been a cancer register in the UK since 1962, but notification is voluntary. Statistics for other diseases may be available from schemes involving hospital activity and GP surveys. In addition, surveys may be undertaken to establish the incidence or prevalence of other specific diseases, and to make estimates of their impact in terms of morbidity. Often such studies involve very different sources of data, and difficulties in linking them contribute to the view that the causes of morbidity represent a 'health care iceberg' (reported in Unwin, Carr & Leeson, 1997). As a result, mortality, or death, is better documented than is the occurrence of the vast array of diseases which people experience (Rothstein, 2001).

The increases and decreases in causes of death or frequencies of specific diseases at one time or another, which are described below, derive from comparisons in rates of death and disease. In order to calculate a rate of occurrence it is necessary to know both the number of individuals who fall into the target category, for example death from lung cancer, and the size of the population from which the fatalities have occurred. This population is described technically as the 'population at risk' (Coggon, Rose & Barker, 1993: 8).

The crude rate of death is a fraction or ratio, in which the total number of deaths during a defined time period forms the numerator, and the average population across the same time period forms the denominator. As the numerator is the number of people who died, if everyone in the population died, the numerator would be the same as the denominator and the ratio would equal 1; the resulting fraction can be no greater than 1. Usually, it is much smaller.

Let us imagine that 6000 deaths from all causes are reported in a city over a year. If the total population averaged 300,000 during that year, the crude death rate for the year would be 6000 divided by 300,000 or 0.02. Although the decimal 0.02 gives the death rate per person, it is customary to multiply this decimal by 1000, thus reporting a crude death rate of 20 per 1000 of the population.

Crude death rates for total populations are of limited use. Mortality rates for specific diseases may be calculated with some confidence from death certificates, but once the 6000 deaths we hypothesised are assigned to almost 400 distinct disease categories, the numbers in each category become quite small. Hence these statistics are usually presented in terms of deaths per 100,000.

The ratio that we have just calculated is described as a *prevalence* rate. A prevalence rate is based upon existing cases that have occurred at a particular time. If the numerator is obtained by counting existing cases on the 1st of July, the resulting fraction is described as a *point prevalence rate*. If the numerator is obtained by counting the number of cases recorded over one year, it is described as a *period prevalence rate*.

Period and point prevalence rates may reveal patterns and raise hypotheses, but new cases are a further important source of information. The number of new cases over a specified time period divided by the population at risk is the *incidence rate*. Some of the issues that arise in determining the denominator or the population at risk when calculating incidence are illustrated in an example provided by Unwin et al. (1997). They noted that it would be relatively straightforward to collect the number of new cases of cancer of the uterus from the cancer register for a city for a year. However, the population at risk is *not* the population of the city for that particular year. First of all, the number of new cases would have to be removed from the total population, so too all males, as they are clearly not at risk, nor are women who have already had a hysterectomy and thus no longer at risk.

One view of the interrelation of prevalence and incidence is presented by Coggon et al. (1993). They describe each new occurrence, or disease incidence, as entering a prevalence pool. They describe two paths out of the prevalence pool – recovery or death. Thus they conceptualise mortality as 'the incidence of death from disease' (p. 10). Recovery carries the potential for further disease episodes and appearance once again in the numerator used to calculate the incidence of disease.

Prevalence and incidence rates can also be compared in terms of their usefulness in framing causal accounts of disease (MacMahon & Trichopoulos, 1996). Incidence rates provide more information about the occurrence of disease as they are gathered closer to the time of disease onset. To maximise this advantage, incidence would ideally be measured as close to onset as possible. As we have noted, death rates are useful because they are collected widely and reliably. MacMahon and Trichopoulos suggest that for diseases with a high fatality ratio and with a short onset/ death interval, death rates may be used as incidence surrogates. Although prevalence rates may have limited usefulness in illuminating causality, they have major implications for resource planning and health care maintenance.

Group membership and epidemiology

In order to understand the 20th-century history of disease in the USA and other industrialised countries, it is necessary to refine crude death rates. Some of the group differences in experience which influence health outcomes are age, sex, race, religion, ethnicity and social class. We begin by looking at age differences in death rates. Table 3.1 shows substantial reductions in mortality across the 20th century for the very young, but little absolute change in mortality rates among middle-aged people. These age group differences illustrate the principle that characteristics that define group membership are associated with different incidences.

Table 3.1   US age-specific death rates 1900–1991 Deaths per 1000

Age group	1900	1930	1960	1991
Under 1 year	162.4	69.0	27.0	9.2
55–64 years	10.2	6.8	3.0	2.2
75–84 years	123.3	112.7	87.5	58.9

Adapted from Rothstein, Table 1, p. 57.

One explanation for the absolute reduction of death among infants and older people is the greater incidence of potentially fatal infectious diseases among the young and the elderly. Improved hygiene, nutrition and vaccination reduced diphtheria, measles, scarlet fever and whooping cough mortality among infants, and improved living conditions reduced mortality from pneumonia and influenza among the elderly.

Examination of changing death rates by age group raises a further issue. This is the changing distribution of age in the population, the denominator or population at risk. During the 20th century, individuals who had escaped the fatal infectious diseases of infancy and childhood aged and eventually developed chronic and degenerative diseases. Mortality from the leading three diseases of middle and old age – heart disease, cancer and cerebrovascular disease – increased from 308 per 100,000 at the beginning of the century to 546 per 100,000 in 1991.

Age-adjusted death rates are produced by statistical procedures to allow comparisons across time periods. By statistically equalising the distribution of age in different populations, the history of specific diseases can be traced using prevalence or incidence rates. It was such age-adjusted death rates that revealed the rise of heart disease in the first half of the 20th century and its subsequent decline in the second half of the century. Rothstein's (2001) thoughts about changes in heart disease mortality are worth considering as they prompt us to think about the major causes of mortality and morbidity:

> Both the upward and downward trends occurred so rapidly that they must have been caused by social and environmental changes, not changes in human biology. ... The trends occurred for both men and women, so that factors that would benefit one sex more than the other cannot be responsible. (p. 63)

Rothstein's comments on the similarity of trends for both men and women is particularly interesting as epidemiological analyses are usually undertaken in a sex-blind fashion, that is to say, results for men and women are pooled and analysed together. As Rothstein did not offer satisfactory causal explanations either for the rise or decline in heart disease mortality from analyses of age or sex group membership, perhaps other group differences, besides age or sex, could provide testable hypotheses.

Searching for explanations

One of the statistics most widely used in trying to understand changes in the occurrence of disease is the standardised mortality ratio usually abbreviated as SMR. SMRs are the measures employed by epidemiologists and public health practitioners to compare the state of health of two or more populations.

To calculate an SMR, the first step is to standardise the observed crude mortality rate of a population in relation to its age structure. As we have already noted, the age structure of intact populations changed markedly in the 20th century as a consequence of the reduction in infectious diseases and improved living conditions. Nowadays fewer younger people die than do older people. You would expect the mortality rate of a town with a large proportion of retired people to be greater than a town with a higher proportion of young families and students simply because it has a higher proportion of elderly residents. An age-standardised mortality rate for either town could be used as the numerator in a ratio in which the denominator would be the predicted age-standardised mortality rate for the general population (say the UK, or often England or England and Wales). This ratio is then multiplied by 100. Once the mortality rates for the two towns were standardised for age, SMRs might be expected to be quite similar.

SMRs greater than 100 represent a specific population which is less healthy (or strictly has a higher death rate, not necessarily the same thing, but in practice often conceptualised as synonymous) than would be expected for its age structure. Conversely, an SMR below 100 indicates a lower-than-predicted death rate for that population and is generally regarded as indicating that those people are healthier than would be expected solely on the basis of their age structure.

Epidemiological studies of mortality and morbidity in England and Wales usually employ occupational groupings to define socio-economic status (SES) but research in the USA has used years of education since the 1960s (Elo & Preston, 1996). In general, SMRs show linear gradients when plotted against socio-economic status (SES) even when standardised for age. The Registrar General's occupational categories define the dependent variables used in the Black report (Townsend, Davidson & Whitehead, 1988) and in most of Wilkinson and Marmot's studies (Wilkinson & Marmot, 1998; Marmot & Wilkinson, 1999). The finding that SMRs for all causes in the UK are about 80 for social class I and about 160 for social class V illustrates the SES effect. Thus, if the social class composition of the town of retirees was markedly higher than that of the town of young people, there would be a difference in SMRs favouring the town of older but more upper-class people. Another way of viewing the SMRs of social class I and V is to note that the average 'risk' of dying prematurely is twice as high if you are in the poorest section of society. We note below that the SES gradient functions more steeply during certain periods in the life span. Although SMRs allow the comparison of health risks by social class, information about the effects of age may be lost if total populations standardised for age are compared.

The social gradient cuts across effects due to age, gender and race. It has proved to be a surprisingly robust predictor of morbidity and mortality and a challenge to intervention strategies. In the next section we look specifically at the effects of sex on health, but before undertaking that examination we consider briefly the influence of age, gender and race on social gradients for mortality and morbidity. There is little doubt that the SES effect is linear for men but the evidence is less clear for women (Elo & Preston, 1996; Matthews, Manor & Power, 1999). In their study of mortality in the USA, Elo and Preston found educational differentials in mortality relating to age, gender and race. SES differentials were greater for working-aged men and women and for men than they were for people over 65 or for women. They also reported a higher overall risk associated with being a black person, rather than a white person, between the ages of 25 and 64 years.

The belief that SES differentials in women's health are smaller than those of men led Matthews and her colleagues (Matthews, Manor & Power, 1999) to re-examine data from the British 1958 birth cohort study. SES measures based upon occupational groupings revealed no statistically significant differences between men and women at ages 23 and 33 years. However, greater inequality among men than women for limiting long-standing illness and respiratory symptoms was revealed at age 33 when SES was assessed by education. This measure revealed greater inequality for women than for men at age 23 in terms of self-rated poor health and at age 33 for psychological distress. This study suggests that the SES effect is modified by age, gender and, indeed, by the measures of SES and morbidity employed.

We reviewed the importance of risk assessment in both professional and lay persons' understanding of health issues in Chapter 2. Relative risk ratios are used to compare the theoretical risk of dying if an individual has a particular characteristic compared to an otherwise similar individual who does not possess that particular characteristic. For example, the risk of dying from coronary heart disease (CHD) may be calculated for a group of people of known social class, age, exercise level, etc., and who are non-smokers. The same calculation can be performed for another group of people who are similar in all known respects *except* for the fact that they are smokers. These are expressed as a ratio, such that the non-smokers (control) group has a theoretical risk given a value of 1.0. Typically, such a calculation gives the relative risk for smokers as about 1.7, that is they are 1.7 times more likely to die from CHD than would people who are similar in respect to all other known risk factors except smoking.

In Chapter 2 we noted Busfield's (2000) concern that medical sociologists, in research designed to explain health, have focused on individual behaviour and that both resources and social interaction have been under-researched. The finding that the relative risk for CHD calculated for having a high cholesterol diet is typically about 1.3 but that for being socially isolated may be as high as 2.8 is consistent with his concern and important evidence deriving from studies of relative risk. The effect holds even when controlling for the fact that socially isolated people may smoke more, drink more (etc.), than do people who have good social networks. Pharmaceutical companies have yet to turn their attention to drugs that might improve social networks. Though such interventions are sorely needed they do not appear to offer a marketing opportunity. Cynically, we may note that statins are widely prescribed. These drugs are believed to reduce cholesterol and hence the risk of CHD, but a risk much smaller than that of social isolation.

In the sections below we examine more closely mortality and morbidity rates associated with significant groups in society and explore the explanations offered for consistent differences. We begin by examining the effects of being male or female, as membership in a sex group has major implications for health. We have already noted that social class influences men and women's health differently. We also note sex groups are not homogeneous.

Sex, gender and health

Sex group membership, alongside age, influences mortality rates. Death rates for the three age groups shown in Table 3.1 are displayed in Table 3.2, but here they are further divided into sex groups. Although sex-specific mortality rates have declined among infants across the century, in both middle and old age this fall has been most pronounced in women. Tables 3.1 and 3.2 illustrate the need for epidemiological research to identify the groups in society that show different rates of death and disease.

Table 3.2   US Age and sex-specific death rates 1900–1991
Deaths per 1000

Age group		1900	1930	1960	1991
Under 1 year:	male	179.1	77.0	30.6	10.2
	female	145.4	60.7	23.2	8.0
55–64 years:	male	28.7	26.6	23.1	15.2
	female	25.8	21.2	12.0	8.7
75–84 years:	male	128.3	119.1	101.8	76.9
	female	118.8	106.6	76.3	48.0

Adapted from Rothstein, Table 2, p. 58.

Before we consider the complex relationship between sex and gender, let us examine Table 3.2 once again. It illustrates one of the clearest results of epidemiological research. By and large, in most societies, females live longer than males. The exceptions to this rule are only Afghanistan, Bangladesh, Bhutan, Djibouti, Iraq, Nepal and Pakistan (WHO, 1994).

A recent study of men in the USA reported not only that women, on average, lived seven years longer than men, but that men had higher death rates for all 15 leading causes of death (Courtenay, 2000). It is particularly noteworthy that, using age-adjusted death rates, the rate for men is twice that for women from heart disease and 1.5 times higher for cancers than that of women. Courtenay reports that almost 3 out of every 4 persons who die of heart disease prematurely, that is, before the age of 65, are men. Although Courtenay records the influence of social indicators, economic and ethnic factors, as well as access to health care, he stresses the importance of gender-specific health behaviours in creating this outcome. We shall be returning to the issue of men and women's health behaviours.

However, when we move from mortality to morbidity, the evidence is less clear. There is a widely accepted stereotype that presents women as sicker than men. Indeed, there is empirical evidence of excess morbidity linked to the specific female reproductive risk (Doyal, 2000; McDonough & Walter, 2001). But the disadvantage experienced by women is not restricted to health. Referencing United Nations Human Development Reports, Eckerman (2000) shows that on both the Gender-related Development Index (GDI) and the Gender Empowerment Measure (GEM) women lag behind men: 70% of the world's poor are women and two-thirds of the world's illiterates are women. Of the world's millions of children who have no access to primary education, 62% are girls. Added to these results are the findings that one-quarter of families are headed by women, yet women obtain only one-tenth of the world's income, own less than one-tenth of the world's property and are found among only 1% of the world's top executives. And finally, as Doyal (2001) notes, around the world, half a million women a year die of pregnancy and in childbirth while '10 times that number are seriously disabled' (p. 1061).

The health hazards of being born female are starkly recorded above, but a moment's thought reveals that they are *not* exclusively biological. Even the most 'biologically' determined findings, reproductive mortality and morbidity, are not evenly distributed around the globe. Death rates are lower in countries where health care is more widely available. The feminine role, that is, women's gender, is socially defined and gender roles vary across and within societies. The mantra that women experience more ill health than do men but that men die younger than do women had become so entrenched that in 1999 Hunt and Annadale (1999) edited a special issue of the journal, *Social Science & Medicine*, in order to examine exceptions to this generalisation.

In order to challenge the immediate occupational effects of gender segregation in employment (cf. Archer & Lloyd, 2002 for a description of gender ghettos in work), Emslie and her colleagues (1999) elicited self-reports of health from full-time employees of a major British bank. Within this restricted population they found that there was no evidence of differences in the reports of men and women concerning physical symptoms and only a slightly larger report of psychosocial malaise by women than by men. Moreover, their standard instrument measuring mental health revealed no sex difference. Indeed, employees' perceptions of their working conditions related more strongly to perceived minor morbidity than did gender. Although this study might be viewed as a special case, another study in the *Social Science & Medicine* special issue, that of Fuhrer and co-research workers (1999), also reported gender similarities from a longitudinal study of middle-aged British civil servants. They noted that 'effects of marital status, social support within and outside the workplace and social networks on subsequent occurrence of psychological distress were comparable for men and women' (p. 83). Nonetheless, they also observed, from baseline measures, that women were at slightly a greater risk of distress (OR = 1.27) than were men.

Macintyre and colleagues (1999) addressed directly the issue of women's alleged over-representation among people suffering from ill health in a paper comparing Scottish men's and women's responses to a standard question about long-standing health problems. The individuals interviewed were either in their late 30s or late 50s. Skilled nurse interviewers followed up a standard question with three additional questions and further probes. The standard question failed to reveal any gender differences, nor were there differences in the mean number of conditions elicited by further questioning. The 'reality' of these self-reports could not be validated as there was no independent measure of health, but an earlier study of the common cold by Macintyre (1993) provides evidence on this issue. In that study, the women who volunteered to take part in an investigation of the common cold reported themselves no more likely to catch cold than did men, but the staff of the research unit believed that women would report themselves more liable to catch cold than were men, and indeed to catch more colds. Even among health research workers, stereotypes are slow to disappear.

We have already noted that different occupational experiences and stereotypes are factors which contribute to the enduring belief that women experience greater morbidity. A further factor is age. Arber and Cooper (1999) have shown that among the elderly there is little difference between men and women in self-assessed health and limiting long-standing illness although women actually experience greater mobility and self-care impairment. Once again social factors affect these sex and gender differences as, on average, women are older, more likely to be widowed and to have had lower occupational status and income than men. As a result of the gender differentiated rates of mortality there are twice as many women as men over 65 years of age. This ratio rises to three times among the over 85-year-olds. Nonetheless, and taking into account the higher level of functional impairment among women, there is no significant difference on a self-assessed report of health using a scale with the points 'good', 'fairly good' and 'not good'.

Despite statistics revealing the reproductive hazards that females endure, we have already noted that the health of women is determined by social factors as well as by biology. In the second wave of feminism in the 1970s and 1980s, a good deal of attention was paid to health issues. More recently social factors have come to the fore in discussions about men's health behaviours (Courtenay, 2000). Courtenay has proposed that the very behaviours that men employ to assert a masculine identity and thus gain power and status may be detrimental to their health. Men in the USA are reported to lag well behind women in adopting an array of health-related behaviours and are more likely to engage in 11 out of 14 risk behaviours than are women. These risk behaviours include smoking, drinking, driving without safety belts, avoiding screening procedures and ignoring symptoms of ill heath. Even among individuals with recognised health problems, men are less likely than women to have sought contact with a doctor. Courtenay brings the argument full circle by asserting that the failure to recognise the consequences of the construction of masculinities perpetuates the belief that the gender difference in mortality is biologically determined. He further asserts that to recognise the poor health status of men in the USA may put at risk the status gained through the unhealthy behaviours employed in the construction of masculinities. If his analysis is valid, the task of changing the health-related behaviours of men is a daunting one.

Social class and inequalities in health

In earlier centuries, when medical interventions were largely ineffective, wealth could influence health and a longer life through better housing, nutrition, sanitation, reduced exposure to contagion, and cleaner water. Advances in biomedical science and clinical practice led to the expectation that if citizens in wealthy nations enjoyed equal access to effective medical care, death rates of rich and poor would soon become more equal. Despite over half a century of health care in the UK, free at the point of need, inequalities in health linked to membership in different groups in society have not only persisted but increased. Explanations are required as the expected improvements in the nation's health have failed to materialise.

As we have already noted, mortality rates decreased sharply in the USA in the 20th century, as they did in most industrialised countries, but group differences, reflecting socio-economic status (SES), only increased across the century in both the USA and the UK (Rothstein, 2001). The significance of SES differences in mortality rates is accentuated by evidence showing that these differences persist across groups divided in terms of age, sex, race and disease.

Cross-national comparisons highlight further the significance of SES. Once industrial or developed nations reach a certain level of prosperity, average national wealth no longer predicts health (Marmot & Wilkinson, 1999; Wilkinson, 1996). Despite life expectancy increasing across the decades in developed countries, it is greater in Greece and Italy than in the USA and Germany, which are considerably richer. The epidemiological transition that sees degenerative diseases and cancer replace infectious diseases as major causes of death also sees the diseases that had previously afflicted rich people become more prevalent among the poor of prosperous nations. Thus the heart disease of businessmen became the cause of working-class mortality. Cross-nationally the correlation between a nation's wealth and health may be small, but within nations the relationship between health and standard of living is well documented.

The classic study of Marmot et al. (1978) demonstrated the importance of social status and the relatively weaker impact of risk factors such as diet, exercise, smoking and drinking, for which individuals have long been exhorted to take individual responsibility. He and his colleagues presented evidence that showed that death from coronary heart disease was a function of occupational status among male civil servants working in Whitehall. Men in the top rank had significantly fewer deaths from coronary heart disease and there was a steady rise in mortality as career grade decreased. This social gradient was only partially explained, (that is between 25 and 40%) by risk factors that individuals might control or those such as height, which reflect genetic endowment.

Medical interventions are by their very nature directed to the individual. An aspect of the medicalisation of health is an approach to health promotion that focuses upon the individual and targets reductions in risk factors such as smoking, drinking and poor diet. The importance of understanding the growing body of evidence that relates disease to social structure and human capital lies in helping to re-focus attention and interventions at a society level (Marmot, 1999; Wilkinson, 1996).

Society and health

Wilkinson (1996) argues that a social science approach is necessary if population health is to be understood. He cites both disease incidence and historical change as evidence for the influence of social and political factors. He buttresses the argument for the influence of social factors by examining the social gradient for the 80 most important causes of death, from the almost 400 contained within the *ICD* system. Roughly 80% of them (76% for women and 83% for men) are more common causes of death among working-class than among middle-class people. The only diseases where middle-class death rates are higher than those of working-class individuals are skin and breast cancers. Wilkinson asserts that the consistency of the tilt in the social gradient across all major disease categories establishes the role of social factors.

Historical comparisons of death rates in Europe in the last three decades of the 20th century furnish further evidence for the influence of social and political processes on population health. Wilkinson (1996 from Watson, 1995) demonstrated that rank ordering the death rates of the countries of Eastern and Western Europe in 1970 revealed considerable overlap between the two blocs. In fact, East Germany had a lower death rate than West Germany and a number of Western European countries had higher death rates than Bulgaria and Romania. By 1990 the rank order had changed dramatically. Using 1990 death rates for men in the same countries and again ordering them from lowest to highest rates, death rates in every former Eastern bloc country were found to be higher than those of every Western bloc country. The former Yugoslavia, which had maintained a position independent of the major blocs, had a death rate that stood between the two. While life expectancy in the Eastern bloc had caught up with that in the West by 1970, there was no further improvement in the East. Thus, by 1990, the gap had widened as population health in the West continued to improve. Evidence suggests that the explanation for the failure of further improvement in the East cannot lie with available health care, economic growth or pollution (Hertzman, 1995). Rather, Wilkinson speculates that were we to understand the socio-political factors that had impeded improvements in health in Eastern Europe, we might have a better understanding of the processes that led to the revolutions of 1989. He believes that a nation's health is an indicator of a society's well-being.

Quality of life

The dialectic of the relationship between health and disease is a recurrent theme throughout this text. In Chapter 2 we examined the definitions of both doctors and lay persons. There is no easy resolution. Bowling (1997) asserts, in the opening chapter of her textbook on measuring health, that:

> Measures of health status need to take both concepts into account. What matters in the 20th century is how the patient feels, rather than how doctors think they ought to feel on the basis of clinical measurements. (p. 1)

Despite this clear statement about the priority of the subjective experience of illness, Bowling acknowledges that most 'health' evidence is presented in terms of five-year survival rates following treatment for disease. This leads back to the measures of mortality and morbidity that we considered at the beginning to this chapter. Acknowledging that 'return to work' is a frequently used non-biological measure of health status employed to assess the effectiveness of a medical intervention, Bowling notes that it is confounded with other non-health variables. These include age, economic and social factors.

Survey research has offered one method for moving beyond the analyses of epidemiologists based upon available statistics. In this domain of self-report, health outcomes are usually measured in terms of functional ability and status. This approach relates the effectiveness of a particular treatment to an individual's ability to carry out the tasks of daily living. The very fact that there may be lacunae in an individual's ability to perform such tasks has led to difficulties in the conceptualisation and description of these deficits. They may be referred to as impairment, disability, handicap or functional dependency, with further implications for the quality of both physical and social life.

WHO (1980) has provided a classification system that has clarified the inter-relationship of these concepts. Impairment stands closest to the biomedical pole but the interruption of such biological functions results in the disability to perform the tasks of daily living. Such handicap can be conceptualised at both a physical and social level. Many people overcome physical disability and function socially with no functional handicap. Despite adequate social functioning, disabled individuals may still be dependent on others to perform essential physical tasks.

Health promotion and quality of life

We propose here that one of the major flaws in health promotion strategy and practice stems from the discipline's epidemiological and public health medicine roots. At the time of writing, the expected lifespan of people born in the UK is over 80 years. As we have detailed elsewhere in this volume, life expectancy and freedom from illness show a marked inverse relationship with both relative and absolute poverty. Yet even the most disadvantaged individuals of the British population stand a very good chance of living to what most people would consider old age. What is less commonly considered in public health terms is the quality of those years of life in terms not solely defined by the absence of illness. Framing quality of life primarily in terms of longevity and the absence of pathology reflects the strongly reductionist viewpoint engendered by the natural and medical sciences. A reductionist approach seeks to explain phenomena by dividing complex entities or organisms (like people) into simple units whose relationships with other simple units may be specified and described. Thus people become bodies, bodies become collections of systems, organs, tissues and ultimately cells.

Thirty years ago, such a tendency was shown to accompany the increasingly scientific orientation of medicine across the 20th century (Riley, 1977), and this tradition has been subsequently inherited by health promotion as a discipline. For example, some people (organisms) develop coronary heart disease. Coronary heart disease occurs when the heart (an organ) ceases to function correctly. The heart's malfunction occurs because of pathological changes in the health of the myocardium and its blood supply (tissues). This in turn is influenced by the biochemistry of the blood (cells), notably by certain forms of cholesterol present in people's (organisms) diet. Thus, the logical way to promote health (defined as preventing disease) is to persuade people to eat less fat: hence the seemingly endless litany of healthy eating advice offered by health promoters. While for many individuals, the value in terms of CHD prevention of reducing dietary cholesterol intake remains controversial, we argue that such an approach actually misses the point.

The view of health espoused by most theorists and practitioners in health promotion defines health in a very different way to that typically adopted by epidemiologists. It follows that the goals that health promotion seeks to achieve should be rooted more in its own definitions and aims rather than those of the medical establishment from which health promotion first emerged and which still, to a greater or lesser extent, manages its activities and priorities.

Perhaps the most important single change in health promotion priorities should be away from reducing the risks of contracting coronary heart disease and cancers and toward investing more, or at the very least equitably, in improving people's emotional and psychological well-being. Blaxter (1995a) asked a large ($n = 9000$) sample of people to describe 'what it is to be healthy oneself'. The results are illuminating for, and an important challenge to, health promoters. Psychological fitness ranked highly across all age groups, and subjects aged over 40 were up to three times more likely to describe psychological well-being rather than physical fitness in their responses. We suggest that given that the absolute importance of self-empowerment and informed choice are generally considered axiomatic in health promotion, then the current balance of funding, personnel and investment in mental health promotion is not only woefully inadequate, but also inconsistent with its own most fundamental principles. Wilcock (1998) notes that:

> if mental well-being is to be attained, [people need] self-esteem, motivation, socialisation, meaning, and purpose as well as sufficient intellectual challenge to stimulate neuronal physiology and encourage efficient or enhanced problem-solving, sensory integration, perception, attention, concentration, reflection, language and memory ... [a balance] between intellectual challenges, spiritual experiences, emotional highs and lows, and relaxation is required ... mental well-being will be enhanced if people ... are able to develop spiritual, cognitive, and emotive capacities; to experience timelessness and 'higher-order meaning' and to adjust their activities to achieve a balanced combination of mental, physical and social use. (p. 102)

The challenge for health promoters here is twofold. Firstly, to be assertive enough and sufficiently well-prepared to argue the case for an apparently radical change in priorities, secondly to be sufficiently creative to develop initiatives which facilitate the personal development that Wilcock describes.

For health promotion to be true to its own philosophy, we suggest that a different approach is indicated. This approach is far from new, yet it is largely ignored by commissioners and managers of health promotion programmes. Nearly a century ago, Hall (1910) noted the vital role of *meaningful activity* in people's lives, suggesting that human activity can be divided into 'changeable periods of work, rest and recreation'. Hall's observation, however, is not a simple exhortation for the carving-up of hours in the day in order to meet the sometimes conflicting requirements of biology and working life; the key concept is that activity should be *meaningful*. Meyer (1922) drew on this point explicitly. Meyer noted the necessity for humans to respond to natural cycles such as night and day, but he went further:

> There are many other rhythms which we must be attuned to: the larger rhythms of night and day, of sleep and waking hours, of hunger and its gratification, and finally the big four – work and play and rest and sleep, which our organism must be able to balance even under difficulty. The only way to attain balance in all this is actual doing, actual practice, a programme of wholesome living as the basis of wholesome feeling and thinking and fancy and interest.

Although Meyer's dated phraseology now seems somewhat quaint or even patronising, his observation has formed the basis for a concept central to much therapeutic practice: that of occupational balance. During the 1960s in the USA, Reilly developed this notion in the treatment of patients at the Neuropsychiatric Institute of the University of California in Los Angeles (Reilly, 1966). Her model aimed to restore patients' life skills within a framework designed around occupational balance. The programme categorised daily activities into three categories. Firstly, tasks related to personal body maintenance, such as eating, sleeping, and hygiene, which Reilly labels *existence*; secondly, work which supplies an income, or *subsistence*; and thirdly, *choosing time*, which may involve leisure and recreation.

We would argue that Reilly's apparently simple approach provides a clue as to how future health promotion activity might be usefully structured. She draws a clear distinction between recreation as relaxation and rest in order to be able to work, and leisure, which she suggests is a period made possible as a result of a satisfying work experience.

Wilcock (1998) has developed many of these ideas into what she describes as an 'occupational theory of human nature'. This theory is founded on three central concepts. Firstly, all people, unless prevented by serious neurological dysfunction, take part in complex, culturally-determined behaviour which arises from their biology, consciousness, cognitive capacity and language. Such behaviour Wilcock labels *occupation*. From this viewpoint, any approach to health promotion which separates mind from body is automatically untenable. Yet despite protestations to the contrary, such a distinction remains a feature of most health promotion activity in the UK: 'mental health promotion' is generally seen as a specialism separate from, for example, healthy eating campaigns. Similarly, CHD prevention programmes rarely address depression, even though the latter may result in behaviours which may then be conveniently labelled as 'risk factors'. From a public health medicine perspective, mental health is still largely viewed in terms of the commissioning of psychiatric services and the prevention of suicide (particularly important, a cynic might argue, if the local league tables are embarrassingly higher than national rates).

It is true that a few initiatives have attempted to bridge the Cartesian gap between body and mind (for example, so-called 'Green Gym' projects), but these are relatively unusual compared to the recent proliferation of smoking cessation classes and the familiar, ubiquitous forests of healthy eating leaflets. In our view, the recognition of Wilcock's first concept is a prerequisite for more effective health promotion programmes, even those which attempt to alter 'risky' behaviour: such behaviour arises from biological and social-psychological roots and is mediated by, and performed within, a cultural setting *which imbues the behaviour with meaning*.

The prognosis for interventions which choose to ignore these facts may be poor. For example, anti-smoking activity which relies unilaterally on appeals to 'reducing risk' (cognition), biology (nicotine replacement therapy), or which fails to acknowledge the identity of smoking as a commonplace and culturally meaningful human activity (as opposed to being simply deviant behaviour) will inevitably meet the very limited success that has characterised such programmes for decades, particularly amongst the young. Health promotion programmes need to go beyond fashionable lip-service to holism: to be effective they must, in our view, not only hold the removal of dualistic notions as a first principle, but they must then actually operate accordingly.

Secondly, Wilcock (1998) suggests that occupation, as described above, is 'indispensable to survival, as well as being an integral part of complex health maintenance systems'. From an occupational perspective, notions of 'health' are closely allied to those suggested by Nutbeam's (1986: 113) definition of 'well-being': 'a subjective assessment of health which is less concerned with biological function than with feelings such as self-esteem and a sense of belonging through social integration'.

Such a view has important implications when planning health promotion activity aimed at reducing inequalities. From this perspective, improving the *lived experiences* of those people who are least advantaged in society should become the aim and the outcome measures of health promotion activity *in themselves*, rather than the ultimate results of inequalities such as increased morbidity and mortality rates.

Clearly, such outcomes are more difficult to measure and compare, partly because they are defined differently by different people. More sophisticated qualitative techniques need to be developed, rather than investing in more and more detailed epidemiological analyses which simply repeat in finer detail what is already known. Yet being more difficult does not warrant the abandonment of such aims and the falling back on familiar measures that are methodologically expedient (but less useful, given that most people in the developed world already avoid making a personal contribution to mortality statistics for over 70 years).

Despite the difficulties, some studies have investigated the salutogenic influence of meaningful activity on individual well-being. The effect of 'occupation' has been reported across a wide range of activities, and has been described in terms of increases in happiness, contentment, peace, life satisfaction, and achievement, often associated with a sense of timelessness. This range of experiences has become collectively known by occupational scientists as 'flow' (Csikszentmihalyi, 1990). Interestingly, some studies have shown that a typical working adult in the USA experiences 'flow' three times more often at work than in free time (Csikszentmihalyi & LeFevre, 1989; Csikszentmihalyi, 1993). Moreover, during these periods, respondents reported significantly greater feelings of happiness, general satisfaction, creativity and concentration. These feelings are not simply pleasantries, but are central to many people's definitions of their own health (Pybus & Thomson, 1985). When asked to define their own concept of well-being, the researchers found that the three most common responses related to having a sound mind, being happy and (only then) a healthy body.

Wilcock's third principle concerns the necessity to recognise the unique and almost infinitely variable nature of human beings resulting from genetic traits and capacities. As the individual matures, this variation is then inseparably combined with cultural influences in a reciprocal relationship which van den Burghe (1989) describes thus:

> Culture can have no empirical referent outside the human organisms that invent and transmit it, and, therefore, its evolution is inevitably intertwined with the biological evolution of our species. (p. 795)

Again, the implications for health promotion programmes are clear: from this perspective, it is meaningless to consider people in groups whose membership is defined by specific behaviours (for example, 'smokers' or 'sedentary'). The meaning of smoking or being sedentary will differ from individual to individual. Similarly, it can be argued that it is less helpful (than might otherwise be imagined) to have target groups for health promotion campaigns such as 'young people' or 'women'. It is perhaps this kind of over-simplification that has in turn driven so many attempts to find 'magic bullets' which will be 'the key' to changing pathogenic behaviours. Examples of such notions abound in popular consciousness, particularly in relation to problem behaviours among adolescents. For example, 'peer pressure', 'self-esteem' and 'assertiveness' have each in turn been the focus of schools-based health education, and all have had very limited effects (Nutbeam et al., 1993). Our view is that models such as that provided by Wilcock offer a richer framework within which to design, operationalise and evaluate activities aimed at improving people's health as opposed to (yet at the same time) reducing their risks of dying from certain prescribed diseases.

FOUR   Social capital for all?

If man is to venture on the rebuilding of Society, he must take nothing for granted. The first question therefore is – With what unit does Nature build the living world? ... it is not the individual; it is the family.

Innes Pearse and Lucy Crocker (1943):
The Peckham Experiment

Early one December, a 14-year-old daughter who had recently developed an acute case of social conscience pressured her father into 'doing something useful' at Christmas. Instead of the traditional over-indulgence in food, alcohol and sloth, she pronounced, her family should attempt to do something to make life a bit more bearable for people not in a position to risk their health in such a fecklessly irresponsible way. So it was that the family of one of the authors (KL) found themselves at seven o'clock one Christmas morning shivering outside the doors of a YMCA building in a run-down part of a once genteel, but now sadly neglected, seaside town. That day nearly 400 people came through the doors. A few were dressed in layers of tatty clothes and carrying the ubiquitous plastic carrier bags, some with dreadlocks, multiple piercings and the essential scruffy dog, fitting most people's idea of 'the homeless' – and some were already fairly drunk. But by far the majority of those attending did not conform to this stereotype. Many were young, lone mothers with babies and toddlers in pushchairs. Many more were elderly, not obviously poor but clearly lonely to a degree that is shameful for a society that fancies itself as humane.

  The author was assigned the task of ferrying people from their homes to the centre. It was then that he met a man we'll call George. George was a tall, thin, elegant man who was impeccably dressed and groomed, living in a large, three-storey house in a quiet, well-maintained Edwardian terrace away from the seafront. He was monosyllabic in response to attempts at conversation and stared vaguely out of the car window all the way to the centre. On arrival, he accepted a cup of tea and sat at a table without speaking. The organisers revealed that George had lived in his house for many years. He brought up three children there until they left home 20 years ago. Five years later, George's wife died, and he had lived there alone ever since. George had almost completely lost the ability to hold a simple conversation because he simply never spoke to anyone for months on end, except on his weekly shopping trip. Perhaps most poignant of all was the fact that the only way the organisers could persuade George to come to the centre for just that day was to describe him as a volunteer helper.

There are thousands of people like George in the UK today. Between 1961 and 2001 the proportion of one-person households rose from 14% to 30% (Office of National Statistics, 2001: 40). Without family support life can be bleak, and so too is the prediction that single adults will constitute well over a third of all households by 2021.

Social capital

Social capital is a term that has become very popular among health promoters over the last decade. Theoretical debate regarding the precise nature and action of social capital is beyond the limitations of this volume, and fuller discussions are widely available elsewhere. However, we believe that there are some interesting associations with social capital (however defined) that provide signposts for the development of innovative health promotion.

Its popular usage as a term has, according to some authors, led to a lack of clarity of exactly what social capital might be. In a recent review of social capital in relation to health promotion, Hawe and Sheill (2000) liken the use of the term to observations made by Bryson and Mowbray (1981) regarding the way in which the word 'community' was used in the 1970s:

> the sentiment echoes [those] who referred to 'community' as a 'spray-on solution' to the complex social problems [of] the late 1970s and early 1980s. ... Substitute the words 'social capital for 'grassroots' or 'community' ... and a present day feeling arises. ... We agree with others who have observed that social capital is on the brink of being used so widely and diversely that its power as a concept may be weakened. (pp. 871–2)

Similarly, Rose (2000: 1421) notes with concern 'the frequency with which social capital is used as a new bottle for old wine'.

Hawe and Sheill (2000) trace the current wide interest in the notion of social capital to the work of Bourdieu (1986), Coleman (1990) and

Putnam (1993; 1995). Although all three authors provide rather similar definitions of social capital, they each suggest somewhat different implications. In synthesising current research literature, Portes (1998: 1) suggests that social capital may be seen as 'the ability to secure benefits through membership in networks and other social structures'. In this formulation, social capital consists of both a relational component of the social organisations to which an individual may belong, and a material component which comprises the resources to which the individual has access as a result of that membership. Thus a relationship of trust and reciprocity exists which Hawe and Sheill (2000: 872) describe as a network which 'oils the wheels of social and economic exchange, reducing transaction costs, allowing group members to draw on favours, circulate privileged information, and gain better access to opportunities'.

Rose (2000: 1422) makes a very valuable contribution in linking social capital and health by defining the former as 'the stock of networks that are used to produce goods and services in society, of which health is one example'. Networks, he suggests, are *relationships between individuals*: 'Whereas an attribute such as religion can be ascribed to an individual, attendance at a parish church involves an individual in a network.'

Rose's use of this particular example may be pertinent to the discussion of religiosity and health found later in this chapter. Rose goes on to note how in earlier times, most networks operated on a face-to-face, informal basis in order to get things done, with the influence of state and large corporate organisations being peripheral to everyday social interactions. Today, the influences of formal organisations are dominant. Rose cites Coleman (1990: 652) and North (1990: 36) in how this change has manifested itself in current society:

> Joint stock companies produce economic growth, the state routinely delivers collective goods such as policing or clean water, and state, market and non-for-profit institutions can provide health insurance and health care. While informal networks continue to exist their products may simply supplement or support formal organisations.

There is much discussion in the literature concerning both what social capital may be and how it may operate to influence health. In particular, Rose (2000) points out that some definitions (e.g. Putnam, 1997) do not allow for a direction of causation to be elicited; that is, does trust and tolerance produce viable networks, or does the existence of effective networks engender behaviour that fosters such positive attitudes and predispositions in individuals?

Rose (2000) reports on a social capital questionnaire developed for use with Russian adults, and his analysis is based on a sample of 1904 individuals in 191 widely dispersed units. Russian citizens were seen as particularly appropriate for such a study because the former Soviet system of health care was collectivist rather than individualist (as in the UK and USA). Thus 'the state, in fact, assumed responsibility for health and individuals were relegated to a more or less passive role' (Cockerham, 1999: 78). Rates of illness throughout the Russian population increased during the latter days of the Soviet Union, and life expectancy failed to rise at the same rate as that for Western Europeans and Americans. Following its collapse in 1991, age-specific mortality rates, especially for men, have been increasing markedly (Eberstadt, 1999). Rose proposed three possible hypotheses. First, human capital (education, social class, education and so on) is the primary determinant of individual health; second, social capital (an individual's informal links with others) is the primary determinant of health; third, human and social capital are each major determinants of individual health.

His results showed that human and social capital both have a considerable independent influence on individual health status. Moreover, when combined, human and social capital explained 29% of the variance in self-assessed physical health and 19.3% of the variance in emotional health of his sample. In the remainder of this chapter, we explore further some of the ways in which elements of social capital may manifest: in family life, spirituality and the natural environment.

Families: influences on health and the quality of life

A holistic model of health promotion requires careful consideration of family life. Clearly, 'family' does not have to imply a mother, father and children. In considering the domestic sphere it is useful to bear in mind a distinction between households and families. Sometimes a household is composed of a 'traditional family' consisting of a married couple and their dependent children; but families/households today include single parents and two parents of the same sex and their children as well as childless couples, unrelated people and individuals living on their own. An emphasis on the family should not be interpreted to mean that we believe that a 'traditional family' formed by a man and a woman in a legally sanctioned relationship is the only legitimate domestic setting. Indeed, in the second half of the 20th century both the nature of marriage and membership in a family underwent major changes.

The Gay community is currently challenging the definition of a marriage. There is demand for reforms that would permit permanent, same sex relationships to be legally recognised and claims that this step would allow Gay persons, in stable relationships, the same social benefits as those enjoyed by heterosexual couples. In the loosest sense, family and household could be interchangeable. The term 'family' might be reserved to describe persons, in any combination of age and gender, who function effectively as a stable unit in terms of offering mutual support and affection, and which provides individuals with meaningful social identities.

Rapidly accumulating empirical evidence demonstrates that stable family life has health benefits for adults and young people as well as for children and adolescents. Indeed, it has been argued that the risks of family breakdown extend to social life, resulting in weakening community integration and increased crime and violence (O'Neill, 2002).

Demographically we note that despite acknowledged risks, the fact is that some 40% of all British mothers will find themselves parenting children on their own at some time (Ermisch & Francesconi, 2000). Lone motherhood brings poverty, including unemployment, lower income, lack of savings and reliance on state aid to single women. In addition lone mothers suffer significantly poorer mental and physical health, and report more difficulties in parenting. Men who have left the mothers of their children also suffer poorer health and are more likely to engage in risky behaviour including heavy drinking, using drugs and engaging in unsafe sex and unsafe driving. About a quarter of non-resident fathers lose contact with their children, having not seen them for a year or more. Morbidity statistics present an even starker picture. Mortality rates of divorced women over 25 years of age are 35–58% higher than are those of similar aged married women, while morbidity rates 70–100% higher are reported for divorced men of 20 to 60 years (ONS, 2001).

The traditional definition of family that we have noted earlier, involving two adults providing a stable household within which children grow and develop, should not be interpreted to imply that we are denigrating older couples, childless couples, single-parents or reconstituted families, wherein step-parents share parenting responsibilities in a continuous manner. Although we may be labelled conservative, with a small 'c', or even reactionary, we report studies undertaken in both the UK and the USA which underline the risks associated with growing up in either single parent or step-parent families. Perhaps the good news is that 74% of British children live in 'traditional' families with their biological parents while another 6% are parented by two adults in reconstituted families. Of the 20% of children living in single adult households, only 2% of children are living alone with their fathers.

Rebecca O'Neill, a research worker at the think tank Civitas, reviewed over 100 studies undertaken in the 1980s and 1990s (O'Neill, 2002). The benefits which she reported of growing up in a traditional family were startling. They emerged even when income was equated across different group types. Divorce, in particular, put children at 50% greater risk of health problems, put them at twice the risk of running away from home and at five times greater risk of suffering abuse. In addition, O'Neill argues that children growing up without their natural father have greater difficulty in relating to peers and adjusting to school. They are more likely to drink, smoke, take drugs and truant. Furthermore, they are more likely to leave school without qualifications and are at three times greater risk of exclusion from school than are children from intact families.

The picture that has emerged from a comprehensive review carried out in the USA is similar (Wilson, 2002). Wilson argues that the recent rise in violence in the USA is a function of the weakness of families. Fathers, he maintains, not only protect mothers and children but provide important role models for their sons. Quoting data from the National Longitudinal Study of Youth, Wilson reported that young people from father-absent homes were twice as likely to be in jail than were young people from intact families. This was true even when income was equated across groups.

Despite the deleterious effects of growing up in a father-absent home, poverty remains one of the most important risk factors working against successful parenting. On the basis of an extensive empirical study of 1750 parents, Ghate and Hazel (2002), of the Social Policy Bureau, have sought to identify avenues for successful intervention in work with families parenting children in poverty. Drawing upon the ecological model of parenting (Bronfenbrenner, 1979; Belsky, 1980), they describe three categories of risk factors which are related to failures in parenting. At a community level they note that impoverished environments typically contain a high proportion of poor families who often experience a multitude of social and environmental problems. At the household or family level, which we have already considered, children are at greater risk if they live with lone parents, or parents who experience low incomes, unemployment, poor housing, and frequent moving. At a third level, the characteristics of individual adults which affect parenting, such as poor coping skills, are recognised as further risk factors. Ghate and Hazel make the important point that there are many families where these risk factors may be identified but where parenting is successful and children develop adequately. They suggest that attention needs to be paid to the protective factors which mitigate the effects of risk. In particular they seek to understand aspects of resilience which buffer households and families against risk according to the ecological model. They cite a review by Belsky (1984) which identified a supportive partner relationship, family and friends who provide support, a close social network and a temperamentally adaptive child as protective factors which can meliorate risk.

Although Ghate and Hazel (2002) suggest that all of the parents in their study could benefit from assistance, they offer practitioners a list of parents whom they describe as 'priority need groups' (p. 236). These are:

- Parents living in the very poorest neighbourhoods
- Parents on the lowest incomes
- Lone parents
- Parents with high malaise scores (inventory which assesses depressive tendencies)
- Parents with 'difficult' children
- Parents with accommodation problems
- Parents with large families.

Although identifying groups at particular risk and in severe need is important, Ghate and Hazel conclude their report by examining the nature of support that parents state that they most need (p. 244). Parental preferences are summarised under these headings:

- Improved accessibility (such as extended opening hours)
- Expansion of services (for example, increasing staff levels)
- Improvement in staff quality and training
- Providing written information for parents to study at home.

These preferences are a mix of social and individual factors and reflect the ecological model which Ghate and Hazel employ.

How are these findings to be interpreted?

A new perspective on social behaviour is provided by contemporary evolutionary psychology. A relevant example is the explanation for child abuse in reconstituted families. Evolutionary psychologists draw attention to the heritable adaptations that have persisted because of the selective advantage which these adaptations provided our ancestors. Hypotheses are then tested by examining the contemporary social life of species whose social lives are structured in ways similar to those of our pre-agricultural forebears. Emlen (1997) has elaborated this approach in order to increase our understanding and improve interventions designed to compensate for the consequences of the disappearance of the extended family and, indeed, the disintegration of the two-parent 'traditional' family. Once again, he considers these changes in family life in terms of increasing child delinquency, school truancy and exclusion, and child abuse. As we have already noted, all of these problems are more frequent in one-parent and step-parent families.

Fundamental to Emlen's analysis is his focus on family genetics. The traditional family of two biological parents and their children, we have already identified, is described as a 'simple' family and an 'intact' family and is differentiated from 'reconstituted' or 'step' families in which an original biological parent has been replaced by an unrelated adult. Intact families are held to function co-operatively and amicably because individuals increase their inclusive fitness (leaving offspring who share their genetic make-up) through investing in their own offspring or those of closely related relatives. Inclusive fitness leads to four predictions about social relations in reconstituted families. Emlen provides evidence from humans in support of each of these.

Firstly, in a reconstituted family the step-parent gains little fitness through caring for unrelated young; hence Emlen predicts that step-parents will offer only minimal care of their new, unrelated stepchildren. Secondly, since there is no biological link step-parents are more likely than natural parents to be sexually attracted to stepchildren and indeed, stepdaughters are at five times the risk of sexual abuse as are biological daughters. Thirdly, among the children themselves there will be less co-operation among half-siblings than among full siblings with whom they share half their genes. Step-siblings are not related genetically and gain no fitness through co-operation. Finally, reconstituted families will be less stable both through children leaving home earlier than in intact families and through the step-parents themselves divorcing. Emlen uses this evidence of stress in reconstituted families to propose five methods to counteract the effects of pre-dispositions that lead to undesirable outcomes:

- Increased awareness of the risks of conflict in reconstituted families
- Appreciation of emotional issues such as guilt
- Recognition of the types of issues that are likely to produce conflict
- Greater awareness of family-oriented traits in choosing replacement mates
- Formal recognition of risks to offspring through a stepfamily arrangement.

These suggestions offer no quick fix but may widen consideration of appropriate interventions.

Although evolutionary psychology provides a new theoretical formulation to long-term problems of social dysfunction, approaches to improving people's participation in local society existed long before it became fashionable for politicians to issue rhetoric about 'tackling social exclusion':

It [The Pioneer Health Centre] is a field for acquaintanceship and for the development of friendships, and for the entertainment by the family of visiting friends and relations. In these times of disintegrated social and family life in our villages, towns and still worse in our cities [1943!] there is no longer any place like this. Nevertheless, man has a long history of such spaces that have met the needs of his social life and the tentative adventure of his children as they grew up: the church, the forum, the market-place, the village green, the courtyard; comfortable protected spaces where every form of fruitful social activity could lodge itself. (Pearse & Crocker, 1943: 69)

Using knowledge about family life raises difficult policy issues. It is obvious that identifying family structure as a powerful influence on health-related behaviour in adolescence can easily be expropriated by unscrupulously reactionary individuals and used as a means to castigate any individual who is raising a child outside the traditional family unit. However, to neglect such influences is to deny the clear need of children and adolescents for stability in their home environments, irrespective of how that environment is constructed, and to disregard the increasing body of evidence of the risks in terms of health-related behaviour that are exacerbated by family breakdown and reconstruction.

Findings such as Emlen's should not be too surprising. Is it so unexpected that adolescents who feel secure and are happier with their self-image have fewer difficulties? Is it really so improbable that children who are brought up by both biological parents in a supportive and caring environment are less likely to exhibit health-related problem behaviours compared to those who live in discord or who have to adjust to a (or a succession of) new parent-figures?

Of course not. Some (even many) might think these findings obvious and self-evident. But to state such findings openly is difficult. Such a view may be unpalatable as well as being unfashionable. Yet despite these difficulties, such a perspective can no longer be dismissed lightly. The models held in affection by 'health promoters' offer only partial explanations for people's behaviour. In order to understand why people do what they do, we need to consider influences that are not under individual control. For academics, there is a need to see beyond the elegant statistical analyses and achieving publication in prestigious journals, despite the undeniable and constant pressure to do so. For practitioners, there is a need to be more cautious about the unquestioning adoption of theoretical models because they appear 'scientific'. Whole people need to be considered, not just sets of attitudes, beliefs and intentions. Whole people also have emotions, hopes, fears, friends, families and cultures. These things may be more difficult to measure but they are no less important. They are also more difficult to attempt to influence in health promotion schemes. But if we adopt such a view and seek to implement them, then those programmes may be better grounded and perhaps more successful.

Spirituality and health

Psychologists regard the domain of spirituality with a powerful ambivalence that reflects the discipline's roots in philosophy. Freud considered religion to be an illusion. Pressurised by the Jewish community into a Jewish ceremony, he married the granddaughter of the Chief Rabbi of Hamburg but was so opposed to its religious tenets that he had considered converting to Protestantism. Palmer (1997) notes that Freud's vitriolic atheism was based on intellectual, formal principles. While Freud maintained his cultural identity in what he described as a 'life-affirming Judaism', he rejected both religious belief and ritual practices. In a letter to Jung on 2nd January 1910, he argued that:

> It has occurred to me that the ultimate basis of man's need for religion is *infantile helplessness*, which is so much greater in man than in animals. After infancy he cannot conceive of a world without parents, and makes for himself a just God and a kindly nature, the two worst anthropomorphic falsifications he could have imagined. (Palmer, 1997, emphasis in original)

Conversely, Jung (particularly later in life) became increasingly convinced that *denial* of a 'spiritual' nature in humanity was indicative of incomplete individuation. Jung (1928, Vol. 7: 173) uses this term to mean a process in which a person:

> [becomes] an 'in-dividual', and, in so far as 'individuality' embraces our innermost, last, and incomparable unique-ness, it also implies becoming one's own self. We could therefore translate individuation as 'coming to self-hood' or 'self-realization'.

Among academics, the struggle for the emergence of psychology as an independent discipline from philosophy has further polarised opinion regarding spirituality and human well-being. In an effort to free itself from what some viewed as an 'unscientific' background, psychology has striven tirelessly to establish itself as 'a science'. This effort has manifested in many ways. Psychology graduates often tend to be more numerate than those from other disciplines in the social sciences; quantitative studies constitute the great majority of the subject's literature; statistical software designed specifically for psychologists is as at least as sophisticated as any developed for engineering or the natural sciences.

Levin (1994) suggests that other factors are also involved. Firstly, while many studies in psychology and epidemiology have reported a link between religiosity and health outcomes, very few of them actually set out to explore this relationship intentionally. Generally, the occasional measure of religiosity has been 'added to the mix' of variables examined in relation to outcomes such as cardiovascular disease and various cancers. Levin notes that:

> Findings bearing on religion-health linkages were then buried in tables, often without comment in either text or abstract, and usually without reference to similar findings from other studies. (p. 1475)

Secondly, Levin suggests that ideological and institutional barriers in medicine have discouraged the dissemination of positive findings. Levin and Vanderpool (1989) summarise the situation thus:

> Western biomedicine, of which epidemiology is a part, is still wrestling with a mind-body dualism that defies consensus; thus for most epidemiologists, any resolution of a mind-body-spirit pluralism is simply beyond consideration. (p. 589)

Despite attitudes in the medical establishment which range from indifference through ambivalence to hostility, several hundred studies concerning the link between religiosity and health do exist. In the late 19th century, John Shaw Billings noted that religious affiliation appeared to operate as a protective factor in differential rates of morbidity and mortality among different social groups (Billings, 1891). A hundred years before Sir Douglas Black embarrassed the government of the day by identifying health inequalities in the UK, the French sociologist Emile Durkheim identified systematic differences in suicide rates between Jews, Catholics and Protestants (Durkheim, 1897). Since then, several reviews of epidemiological studies have been produced which have yielded similar results. One of the earliest of these, by Jenkins (1971), is notable because of its publication over 30 years ago in the *New England Journal of Medicine*, which prepared the way for many others in 'mainstream' medical journals. Yet perhaps the most controversial work appeared 17 years later in the *Southern Medical Journal* (Byrd, 1988), in which the author reported the apparently positive results of prayer on coronary care outcomes. The study resulted in so much controversy that it provoked a flurry of editorials and essays in journals ranging from the *Journal of Family Practice* to *Social Science & Medicine*.

Levin (1994) traces the more recent literature in this field and notes that studies of religion and health have appeared in most leading medical journals including the *Journal of the American Medical Association*, the *Lancet*, the *American Journal of Public Health* and the *American Journal of Epidemiology*.

Given the long and respected list of publications which have reported at least associations between spirituality and health, the question arises as to why the widespread dissemination of such data has not resulted in any meaningful response from health promotion workers. We would suggest that the answer may involve a failure to distinguish between organised, formal religion and human spirituality in general. The understandable reticence of statutory funding bodies to become involved with religion and its associated social and political complications has, in our view, resulted in an extensive and important area of human experience remaining in receipt of very little attention from health promotion theorists and virtually none from practitioners.

Yet such reticence is hardly evidence based. In an early review of such studies, Levin and Schiller (1987) concluded that generally speaking, religiosity, however operationalised, seems to exert a salutary effect on health, regardless of the outcomes or diseases or types of rates which are examined. In addition, Levin and Schiller reported two other major findings. When comparing religious groups, there appears to be relatively lower risk of illness among adherents to more behaviourally strict religions or denominations. For example, Mormons, Seventh-Day Adventists, Orthodox Jews and clergy of all faiths appear to be at lower risk of morbidity and mortality than do more behaviourally 'liberal' people. Secondly, within religious denominations, there is a trend towards better health, lower morbidity and lower mortality rates among people with higher levels of religiosity. Rates of religious attendance are inversely linked to a strikingly wide range of illnesses, including hypertension, trichomoniasis, cervical cancer, tuberculosis, neonatal mortality and many other conditions, as well as to overall mortality rates. Levin and Schiller noted that this relationship is found in all faiths: their review included all major religious groups, as well as Sephardic Jews, Benedictine monks, Baptist clergy, Adventists, Mormons and Zen Buddhists. Moreover, this relationship persisted however the notion of 'level of religiosity' was operationalised.

Clearly, such findings need to be assessed critically. Levin argues that it is necessary to consider a number of distinct issues before any real relationship between religiosity and health may be viewed to be likely. Firstly, can such an apparent relationship be due solely to chance effects or to biased studies? Levin suggests that such causes alone are unlikely for several reasons. Firstly, hundreds of published studies overwhelmingly report statistically significant positive associations between religiosity and health. Most of these are epidemiological studies of entire populations or of randomised samples. Secondly, there has been considerable diversity in the design of the studies involved, including prospective, retrospective, cohort and case-control studies, in studies both of children and of adults. Moreover, many of these studies have been multi-ethnic in nature, including samples of US white and black Protestants, European Catholics,

Indian Parsees, Zulus from South Africa, Japanese Buddhists and Israeli Jews. Thirdly, Levin's review identified consistent results from studies drawn from a 50-year period between the 1930s and the 1980s. Finally, such studies have been applied to a wide range of physical conditions, including both self-limiting acute illnesses and fatal, chronic diseases. Consistent associations also have been noted in relation to illnesses with long, short or absent latency periods between exposure, diagnosis and mortality. Thus it seems improbable that any observed relationship between religiosity and health can be explained solely in terms of chance or bias effects.

Secondly, it is possible (and perhaps likely) that people who hold strong religious beliefs may behave differently to others, particularly in terms of the health-related behaviours that are the traditional targets of health promotion activity: smoking, excessive alcohol use, drug misuse, an over-rich diet, lack of exercise and liberal sexual behaviour. Yet the congruence of many religious and health-related behaviours may suggest that compartmentalisation into 'religious' and 'health-related' behaviours is artificial.

Thirdly, heredity may be an influence. Some religious communities rarely marry outside their own faith, a practice which may serve to maintain a 'healthy gene pool', thus reducing the prevalence of certain diseases in those groups. There is some evidence to support this suggestion. For example, a high incidence of Tay Sachs disease has been reported among Ashkenazi Jews, as has a similarly high incidence of hypercholesterolaemia among Dutch Reformed Afrikaaners, and of sickle cell anaemia among (predominantly black) US National Baptist Convention members. By contrast, there is a correspondingly low incidence of sickle cell anaemia among (predominantly white) US Southern Baptist Convention members. Clearly, these differences are likely to be due to the genetic characteristics of different religious groups, rather than theological differences; however, such characteristics do not account for the effects of changes in religious affiliation, nor for the marked overall effect of religiosity versus non-religiosity.

Fourth, it is conceivable that frequent religious involvement has salutogenic 'side-effects' which are psychosocial in origin. Many possible mechanisms have been considered (independent of considerations of religiosity) and some of these are discussed elsewhere in this book. Perhaps the most extensively investigated is social support, both in material and practical terms. However, other studies have suggested beneficial effects of possessing a sense of belonging and of order. Antonovsky (1979; 1987) developed the notion of Sense of Coherence (SOC), which he suggests has three component factors, namely comprehensibility (the extent to which an individual sees his/her life as meaningful and comprehensible), manageability (the extent to which problems are seen as manageable) and meaningfulness (the degree to which life is seen as having some kind of meaning).

Clearly, religious belief and ritual may serve to engender a sense of coherence among practitioners which is entirely congruent with Antonovsky's components of SOC. On the other hand, it is also possible that religiosity may have an opposite effect. The dogma associated with some religious traditions manifestly encourages guilt, low self-esteem and doubt, in addition to a social ordering which many people would find oppressive.

Nevertheless, a number of studies have explored Antonovsky's concept of SOC, and have noted a relationship between a high SOC and a low level of illness. For example, Bäckman (1990; 1991) reports results from two Finnish studies where items from Antonovsky's scale were related to good health although, the direction of this relationship is unclear as both of these were cross-sectional studies. Nevertheless, longitudinal studies have also reported a relationship between SOC and both physical and mental health (Dahlin et al., 1990; Kalimo & Vuori, 1990; 1991).

From a health promotion perspective, it is important to note that most of these studies have approached SOC from a psychological frame of reference. Antonovsky, by contrast, views SOC as a social concept; thus SOC grows among people brought up in a socio-economically stable environment with *clearly defined norms and values* (such as among religious groups). Plainly, given Antonovsky's definition, a reasonable beginning for any analysis of the distribution of SOC would be those commonly-agreed demographic variables known to influence health status: sex, age and social class.

Lundberg and Nyström Peck (1994) explored the relationship of SOC to demographic variables and to ill health in the Swedish population. In a sample of 3872 people aged 25–75, they found that the risk of circulatory problems was 80% higher in respondents with low SOC, while such people were at a 300% increased risk of psychological problems. When all other known risk factors were controlled, individuals with low reported SOC remained at a 50% increased risk of circulatory disease and a 250% increased risk of psychological distress. Lundberg and Nyström Peck conclude that the observed relationship is likely to be causal, that having a high SOC may be protective against circulatory and psychological problems, and importantly, that SOC is both internally and externally determined.

Fifth, Levin considers the psychodynamics of belief systems, religious rites and faith, particularly in relation to placebo effects. The combination a sense of purpose, the easing of fear and uncertainty, and a strong belief in the salutary effects of religion may all combine to produce health-enhancing results.

Yet the link between religiosity and health may still not be causal. Hill (1965) proposed a list of nine qualities in a relationship, the presence of some of which at least may be considered supportive of causality. Levin (1994) employed this framework to consider the relationship of religiosity and health outcomes, and found seven of these criteria (strength, consistency, temporality, a biological gradient, plausibility, coherence, and analogy) to be met. While one of the remaining criteria, experimental evidence, is provided by Byrd's (1988) study of prayer on coronary care outcomes, the study remains controversial, and differs from other studies in that it involved people who prayed for them, as well as other patients praying themselves. The final criterion, specificity, requires the independent variable to have an effect on a specific dependent variable (in this case, on specific disease). As religiosity appears to have an effect on a wide range of health-related outcomes, his criterion is not met by definition, rather than by weakness of the association.

Of course, it is entirely possible that a combination of many factors may explain some of the apparently salutogenic effects of religiosity via psycho-neuroimmunological pathways. However, if this is true, Levin's argument elegantly articulates the pointlessness (in our view) of 'explanation' without translating such findings into intervention:

> For example, while there is greater mortality among lonely widows and single men, it is hardly sufficient to say that this is fully explained by psycho-neuroimmunologic factors, even though the process of mortality is reducible to certain physiological and biochemical events. Granting explanatory primacy to one particular level of the human system (cultural, social, psychological, organ systems, cellular, molecular, etc.) is arbitrary; human biology is itself 'explained' by the activity of molecules and ultimately, to paraphrase Democritus, everything is just atoms and empty space. Yet no-one would suggest that research in atomic physics will yield the best approach for improving the life expectancy of lonely or bereaved people. (Levin, 1994: 1477)

Whether or not the nature of an undeniable relationship between religiosity and health becomes clarified by future research is, in our pragmatic view, irrelevant. Historically, some form of spirituality may be seen as a basic human characteristic, which manifests itself in culturally moderated forms. Moreover, its effects on health outcomes appear to be very pronounced. For example, Comstock and Partridge's (1972) study showed infrequent church attendance to carry a relative risk ratio of 3.9 for certain diseases. By contrast, King and Locke (1980) report standardised mortality ratios among the clergy as low as 9 for some causes of death. If only a fraction of these results were attributable solely to spirituality, they would remain effects comparable in magnitude with the more familiar targets of health promotion activity.

To operationalise 'spiritual health promotion' is a complex and difficult task, which in practicality cannot be separated from issues of social inclusion, community development and political considerations. Moreover, such a suggestion is likely to be met with all manner of scepticism and obstacles, both real and imagined. Nevertheless, in our view, interventions which encourage or facilitate the expression of spirituality are likely to yield at least the same benefits as more conventional health promotion 'initiatives'.

Nature and health

The relationship between natural environments and improvements in health status is the focus of an emerging body of research. Until relatively recently, environmental health, as an academic discipline, tended to concentrate on the effects of exposure to hazards such as toxic chemicals, microbiological pathogens and radiation, in addition to atmospheric and water and noise pollution. As a consequence, environmental health as a professional occupation has (quite rightly) devoted much of its attention to the prevention of diseases related to these risks. Across the UK, environmental health teams are employed to safeguard the public from exposure to toxins, food poisoning and workplace hazards. This activity is supported by appropriate legislation and considerable powers are invested in environmental health professionals.

The positive, salutogenic effects of human exposure to healthy natural environments is supported by a growing body of evidence. Frumkin (2001) reviews some of this evidence and suggests that those working to promote health should move their attention 'beyond toxicity' (p. 234) to consider the positive effects of environmental exposure. He draws heavily on the work of the celebrated biologist and ecologist Edward Wilson (Wilson, 1984; Kellert & Wilson, 1993). Wilson developed what has become known as the 'biophilia' hypothesis, in which he suggests that human beings are innately attracted to other living organisms as a result of the evolutionary advantages found in acquiring sensitivity to the natural environment. Frumkin supports this view. Wilson argues that people only very recently began to live lives that are insulated from the environment. If the last 65 million years of primate evolution were compressed to a human lifetime of 70 years, then *Homo sapiens* first settled into villages eight months after their 69th birthday. Frumkin notes that from an evolutionary perspective, it is unsurprising that modern humans have a deep-seated connection with the natural world. As Frumkin notes:

> From an evolutionary perspective, a deep-seated connection with the natural world would be no surprise ... we have broken with long-established patterns of living rather late in our life as a species. (2001: 236)

From a 'biophilic' view, patterns of adaptation cannot be expected to be ephemeral, but will continue to influence human lives, even in that tiny proportion of people who have existed for one or two generations in wholly urban environments.

The notion that a relationship with nature may in some way promote health is a common one with a long history, and Frumkin observes that it may be found in philosophy, art and popular culture from ancient Greece to the 19th-century New England transcendentalists such as Thoreau and Emerson (cf. Nash, 1982; McLuhan, 1994; Mazel, 2000; Murphy et al., 1998). In addition, the expression of a need to escape to wild, unspoiled places is so anecdotally common among modern urban people as to be an almost universal characteristic. Yet it is possible that such a need is merely an aesthetic response rather than one based on biological necessity. In examining empirical and epidemiological evidence for any reliable health-promoting effects of the natural environment, Frumkin (2001) considers four categories, or domains, of nature contact – animals, plants, landscapes and wilderness experience.

Animals

There is considerable evidence linking contact with animals and human health. Frumkin (2001) suggests that it is very likely that the presence of animals or pets may help to reduce stress responses in humans generally. The therapeutic use of animals in psychiatry is now well-established (Draper, Gerber & Layng, 1990).

Anderson, Reid and Jennings (1992) conducted a study of nearly 6000 patients in an Australian cardiovascular disease clinic. Male patients who owned pets had statistically significantly lower systolic blood pressure, serum cholesterol and triglycerides than did men who did not own a pet. These differences did not appear to be related to differences in exercise levels (for example, walking a dog), dietary habits, social class or other confounding factors. Similarly, Friedmann and Thomas (1995) followed up 369 myocardial infarction survivors for 1 year. The 1-year survival rate of patients who were dog-owners was six times that of patients who did not own a dog.

Such retrospective studies are supported by others with prospective designs. Serpell (1991) studied 71 adults who had recently acquired pets, and compared them with a control group who did not have contact with animals. One month after acquiring a pet, the owners showed a statistically significantly reduced incidence of minor health problems, which some owners maintained throughout the 10 months of the trial. In a similar study conducted in the USA, Siegel (1990) divided nearly 1000 Medicare patients into those who owned a pet and those who did not. The pet owners were found to have fewer doctor consultations than did the non-pet owners. Moreover, stressful life events were associated with more doctor consultations among non-pet owners but not among pet-owners, suggesting that pet ownership may help mediate stress. Allen (1997) exposed individuals to a stressful stimulus in three conditions: alone, in the presence of a friend, and with their dog present. In each case, Allen measured individuals' autonomic responses. The stress responses were marked when the subjects were alone, and even more marked when in the presence of a friend; however, the presence of a dog reduced, to a statistically significantly level, the stress response.

In an earlier study, Katcher and colleagues (Katcher, Segal & Beck, 1984) had measured the effects of animal presence on patients who were about to undergo oral surgery. They were randomly assigned to one of five conditions: 30 minutes looking at an aquarium, with or without hypnosis; 30 minutes looking at a picture of a waterfall, with or without hypnosis; and a control group who were simply asked to sit quietly for half an hour. During the surgery, the patients' comfort and relaxation were independently rated by the patients themselves, the surgeon and the investigator. The patients who had previously looked at the aquarium were the most relaxed, irrespective of whether or not they had been hypnotised. Of the patients who had looked at the waterfall picture, only those who had been hypnotised approached the levels of relaxation of the aquarium group; those who had looked at the waterfall but had not been hypnotised had relaxation scores as low as the control group.

Plants

Plants are Frumkin's second domain of nature contact. Lewis (1996) has described the long and established role of horticultural therapy in the treatment of mental health problems. Its use is widespread, ranging from community-based programmes for people with learning difficulties to prison rehabilitation schemes.

Conversely, the aesthetic impoverishment brought about by forced deprivation from contact with plants (caused by hospitalisation) and subsequent positive psychological effects following a visit to a hospital garden has been powerfully described by Sacks (1984; cited in Frumkin, 2001):

I had not been outside in almost a month ... *some essential connection and communion with nature* was re-established after the horrible isolation and *alienation* I had known. *Some part of me came alive* when I was taken into the garden, which had been starved, and died perhaps without my knowing it.

Similarly, Yi (1985) describes the effects of her first visit to a hospital greenhouse in New York's Rusk Institute during her stay following a stroke at the age of 29:

It was when I walked through that building perfectly quiet, filled with green and growing plants and the sweet smell of healthy soil that my anxiety began to ebb away. In its place came a tranquillity *I had not experienced since the day of my stroke.*

(cited in Frumkin, 2001: 237)

The italics in the foregoing quotations are our own, and indicate what we believe to be powerfully descriptive statements from Sacks and Yi about the ways in which they assessed their own health status during the process of their rehabilitation following serious injury and illness. As such they are potent examples of how a change is required in the kind of evidence employed in determining health promotion priorities. We suggest that in order to shift from simply preventing certain diseases to truly promoting health, there needs to be a greater acceptance of the use of qualitative methodologies, and the validity of narrative accounts generally, in understanding what is important to people's subjective experience of health and a greater application of such findings in deciding on the content of health promotion programmes.

Landscape

Returning to Wilson's hypothesis, it may be possible that our preference for, and the therapeutic effects of, landscape may also be evolutionary in origin. Wilson suggests that if any organism, including humans, selects the correct habitat, its life (and hence chance of survival) is easier. Frumkin (2001) offers a range of evidence that people's aesthetic preferences are generally consistent with habitats which would be the most conducive to survival in the wild, and that these preferences are consistent across North American, European, Asian and African cultures (Hull & Revell, 1989; Purcell et al., 1994; Korpela & Hartig, 1996). Yet these preferences are not merely aesthetic whims: viewing such landscapes has been shown to induce relaxation (Ulrich, 1993), decrease fear and anger and enhance positive affect (Honeyman, 1992), and improve mental alertness, attention and cognitive performance in formal psychological testing (Hartig, Mang & Evans, 1991; Cimprich, 1993; Tennessen & Cimprich, 1995).

Further evidence for the health-promoting effects of landscape is found in the rehabilitation literature. Ulrich (1984) compared the records of treatment outcomes for cholecystectomy patients in a Pennsylvanian hospital over a 10-year interval. Postoperatively, such patients were assigned effectively randomly to rooms which either had a view of a group of deciduous trees or a brick wall. Restricting data to summer months when the trees were in leaf, Ulrich reviewed the patients' length of hospitalisation, need for anxiolytics and analgesia, and occurrence of minor postoperative complications. Patients who recovered in rooms with tree views had statistically significantly shorter hospitalisation periods, and needed statistically significantly less analgesia than did patients whose rooms looked out on a brick wall. Heerwagen (1990) used self-report measures of anxiety and blood pressure among patients awaiting dental treatment in a similar study. Half the time a large mural of a landscape scene was displayed on a wall in the waiting area, while the mural was removed the rest of the time. On the days when the mural was in place, patients' self-reported anxiety and blood pressure was lower than on days when it is was absent.

We suggest that while the overall effect of such changes on patients' cardiovascular health may be limited, the effect on regular attendance, and thereby on dental health, might be considerable. What is required is firstly a willingness to give these kinds of studies serious consideration, and secondly to have sufficient insight to make such connections in terms of promoting health.

Wilderness experience

Finally, we consider the effects of entering and spending time in natural landscapes rather than simply viewing them, an activity known in the USA as 'the wilderness experience'. Much of the literature in this area concerns the effects of outdoor experience on mental health. Early descriptions of so-called 'wilderness therapy' reported positive outcomes for people with mental health problems (Jerstad & Stelzer, 1973; Plakun, Tucker & Harris, 1981; Witman, 1987; Berman & Anton, 1988). Similarly, benefits have been reported among emotionally disturbed children and adolescents (Hobbs & Shelton, 1972; Marx, 1988; Davis-Berman & Berman, 1989); among bereaved people (Moyer, 1988; Birnbaum, 1991); and among rape and incest survivors (Levine, 1994). However, benefits are also reported among adolescents with cancer (Pearson, 1989); children with severe renal disease (Warady, 1994); adults with post-traumatic stress syndrome (Hyer et al., 1996); and addictive disorders (Bennett, Cardone & Jarczyk, 1998).

Frumkin (2001) proposes that, taken together, this growing body of evidence has implications for research and intervention. In terms of research, he spells out explicitly the theme that recurs consistently throughout this book: the need to move away from illness prevention towards health improvement. Frumkin writes:

We need a research agenda directed not only at exposures we suspect to be unhealthy, but also at those we expect to be healthy, and at outcomes that reflect not only [reducing] impaired health, but also enhanced health. If people have regular contact with flowers or trees, do they report greater well-being, better sleep, fewer headaches, reduced joint pain? ... Do gardens in hospitals speed recovery ... what kinds of contact with nature have the greatest efficacy and cost effectiveness? (2001: 238)

We would argue that the evidence available for the salutary effects of natural environments on health is now sufficient to warrant serious consideration by those who plan and implement health promotion programmes. Encouraging people to look after an animal, to garden or simply to spend time in the natural environment may not have such obvious appeal as hectoring the sedentary to join a gym, but it may prove to be more therapeutic and hence be met with higher adherence, and even result in measurable health benefits.

FIVE   Reasoned Action?
More theory than evidence

We have lost the art of living; and in the most important science of all, the science of daily life, the science of behaviour, we are complete ignoramuses. We have psychology instead.

D.H. Lawrence

Obscurantism is the academic theorist's revenge on society for having consigned him or her to relative obscurity – a way of proclaiming one's superiority in the face of one's diminished influence.

David Lehman

During the 1980s and 1990s, nursing practice in the UK became influenced by a number of models, frameworks and theories. These formulations, quite laudably, attempted to provide a theoretical grounding for nursing practice. In addition, they encouraged clinical nurses to become less focused solely on the patient's illness, and more on the person being cared for as a whole.

One day, the first author found himself a day patient in a large general hospital, awaiting minor surgery to one hand. The nurse dealing with his admission went through the most exhaustive checklist imaginable. The procedure was based fairly tightly on Nancy Roper's model of care, perhaps one of the most influential of such theoretical frameworks. Despite being completely healthy other than for a 'trigger finger', the patient was asked about his ability to climb stairs, cook, wash, feed himself, express his sexuality and earn a living. This process took somewhere in the region of a quarter of an hour, and included a discussion of whether he might like to talk to a social worker, and the possibilities of 'meals-on-wheels' following discharge.

> The operation passed without incident, and the patient awoke and was offered tea. Apart from having one hand wrapped in padded bandages to the elbow, and his arm in a high sling tied around the neck, all was well. After a perfunctory check of his blood pressure, the same nurse put her head around the curtains, chirped brightly, 'You can go home now', and disappeared, never to return.
> Presumably, Roper's model never told her how difficult it is to tie shoelaces with one hand.

As an emergent discipline, health promotion has long been preoccupied with two issues: firstly, to find a 'key' to altering people's pathogenic behaviours such as cigarette smoking, alcohol misuse and physical inactivity. Secondly, that it should do so by methods based on 'scientific' principles. To these ends, health promoters have turned to the social sciences for inspiration. The result is that a number of social-psychological models have become highly influential in shaping health promotion programmes, both in the UK and elsewhere. This chapter reviews the most important of such models, and considers their limitations when used as a basis for 'real-life' health promotion initiatives. The terms 'model' and 'theory' are used here interchangeably.

Four major theories are discussed:

1. The Health Belief Model (Rosenstock, 1966)
2. Subjective Expected Utility theory (Edwards, 1954)
3. The Theory of Reasoned Action (Fishbein & Ajzen, 1975; Ajzen & Fishbein, 1980)
4. The Stages of Change Model (Prochaska & DiClemente, 1982b).

A variant of the third of these, known as the Theory of Planned Behaviour (Ajzen & Madden, 1986), is also considered.

Whilst there are important differences in both their premises and operationalisation, all four of the models display much commonality. The Health Belief Model has arguably been more important historically than Subjective Expected Utility (SEU) theory, although it is based on very similar principles. Moreover, the Theory of Reasoned Action was developed directly from SEU theory. All of these models may thus be viewed as having a common core, being variants of expectancy-value approaches to explaining health-related behaviour. The Stages of Change Model (Prochaska & DiClemente, 1982b) was derived from the psychotherapy literature and has been adopted widely in UK health promotion programmes, particularly those concerned with cigarette smoking. In each case, therefore, the theory is first described, and its most relevant applications are reviewed.

The models are then evaluated in terms of their relative strengths and limitations in explaining health-related behaviour. In the case of the Theory of Reasoned Action, and its recent development, the Theory of Planned Behaviour, the models' similarity is such that many criticisms of one may be applicable to the other.

The Health Belief Model

The Health Belief Model (HBM) dates from the early 1950s and was described by Rosenstock (1966), Becker (1974), and Maiman and Becker (1974). It was originally developed by Hochbaum in the US Public Health Service in order to examine reasons for participation, or otherwise, in genetic screening programmes (e.g. Rosenstock, 1974).

According to the HBM, the likelihood of an individual taking a given health action is proximally determined by the sum of perceived benefits and perceived barriers to that action, together with the perceived threat of the consequences of an action (for example, the risk of lung cancer from smoking or heart disease from inactivity). These variables are said to be influenced by other factors, both internal, 'modifying variables', such as age and education, and external, such as media campaigns or advice from health professionals. The level of perceived threat is held to be determined initially by an individual's perceived susceptibility to, and his/her perception of, its seriousness.

During the 1970s and 1980s, the Health Belief Model underpinned a wide range of health promotion activities, including immunisation (Aho, 1979; Cummings, Jette & Brock, 1979), blood pressure screening (King, 1982) and wider preventive behaviour (Oliver & Berger, 1979). Later applications include smoking during pregnancy (Maclaine & MacLeod Clark, 1991). In their study, qualitative analysis of interviews with pregnant women showed that, in support of the HBM, women's views were polarised into groups of high and low susceptibility with regard to the deleterious effects of their smoking. Further, those with high susceptibility beliefs also reported high levels of guilt concerning their smoking. This more recent study is of particular interest in that despite qualitative methodology employing a wide-ranging interview schedule, participants, identified factors which are very similar to features of the model as salient influences in their own decision-making processes.

Michie, Marteau and Kidd (1990) also applied the HBM in pregnancy, in a study concerned with attendance at antenatal classes. Among a range of factors, including sociodemographic variables such as age, social class, country of origin, income and parity, the best predictors of attendance were the perceived costs and benefits of attending. However, it should be noted here that this study also found intention at 28 weeks of pregnancy to be highly predictive of subsequent attendance. Intention is not an original component of the HBM, but has more recently been imported into the model as a result of the influence of other models such as those described below.

Other applications of the HBM have established links with the literature concerning concordance with advice from health professionals. In an early review of this work, Becker and Rosenstock (1984) reported that perceived benefits and costs were significant predictors of behaviour in 18 out of 19 studies. In a later study, MacLeod Clark, Haverty and Kendall (1990) examined the role of trained nurses in smoking cessation interventions, using a framework based partly on the HBM and partly on the nursing process, resulting in very favourable rates of cessation at one year follow-up.

Most studies utilising the HBM have been cross-sectional. This is problematic in that data on beliefs and behaviour are collected at the same time. Whilst the studies have shown strong correlations between beliefs and behaviour, it is difficult to judge whether beliefs produce behaviour or vice versa as there is evidence to show that individuals sometimes rationalise their beliefs to fit with their behaviour (McKinley, 1972). One exception is the early work of Calnan (1984), in a study of participation in breast cancer screening programmes. In this research, analyses were based on prospective studies in which the information concerning beliefs was measured before information on behaviour. Calnan found that whilst the HBM variables were among the best predictors of attendance at each of the services, the variance explained by them was small; the best predictor of attendance was, as in the study by Michie et al. (1990), intention. It is of note that the other variables assessed by Calnan were wide-ranging in nature and included locus of control, self-esteem, social support and normative pressure. However, the latter is described in the study as being 'only measured very crudely' and Calnan goes on to state that such findings '... support Fishbein and Ajzen's (1975) proposition that a specific behaviour is determined by that person's intention to perform that behaviour' (p. 829), and points to the somewhat more comprehensive assessment of normative beliefs in the Fishbein and Ajzen model discussed below.

Pederson, Wanklin and Baskerville (1984) also linked concordance and the HBM in a study of cigarette smoking. They found that HBM variables could be used to explain, albeit only partially, why some individuals stopped smoking when advised to do so by their physicians. However, they found that many smokers held strong health beliefs about smoking's deleterious effects, but did not attempt to stop. Further, such discrepancies between beliefs and behaviour could be accounted for by their additional measures of 'reasons for smoking'. The authors conclude that:

constructs from the HBM ... do not function completely in isolation in determining health behaviour ... the results of this study suggest that the patients' response to advice may depend on the interaction of health beliefs and other variables such as 'reasons for smoking'. (p. 579)

Their paper clearly illustrates the limitations of the HBM in predicting behaviour. It also indicates a major area of weakness common to all similar models: 'reasons for smoking' are themselves composed of smokers' beliefs about smoking which do not fit into the model's somewhat circum-scribed categories. Calnan (1984) also draws attention to an extension of this point:

evidence from recent studies shows that lay models of health and its control do not match up with those of the HBM. ... [the HBM] assumes that the general public as a whole shares the same definitions of health, and [that] this definition is congruent with official medical definitions. (p. 830)

Moreover, as Blaxter and Paterson (1982), Williams (1983) and Calnan (1987) have demonstrated, not only do lay beliefs about health vary with socio-economic status, but lay definitions may also differ markedly from medical ones.

Several authors have identified further weaknesses in the use of the HBM in explaining health behaviour. An important example concerns the fact that the model makes no assumptions as to how the variables combine to influence the behaviour in question. The result has been described as 'a collection of variables rather than a developed theory' (Sutton, 1987: 367) and 'the eclectic nature of the HBM which in its extended form embraces a wide range of factors with no coherent theoretical framework' (Calnan, 1984: 829).

This apparently arbitrary selection of variables and the atheoretical nature of their combination has been described by Wallston and Wallston (1984) as the 'Ptolemic Effect' (analogous to the increasing number of 'epicycles' invoked in early geocentric cosmologies to explain the apparent paths of planetary bodies) in which ever-increasing numbers of variables do not necessarily improve prediction.

Further shortcomings of the HBM have been noted by Sutton (1987). Importantly, the model does not include any variable representing an indi-vidual's decision to perform a given behaviour. Significantly, in studies where such a variable has been included, the model's ability to predict behaviour improves somewhat (Calnan, 1984). Further, the HBM empha-sises perceived susceptibility and severity with respect to a single conse-quence, ignoring other relevant consequences which may be positive or negative. For instance, a woman who smokes during her pregnancy may perceive negative outcomes (e.g. risk to her baby) and positive outcomes (e.g. reduced irritability and increased coping ability) at the same time. In an attempt to produce a parsimonious model consistent with a 'scientific' paradigm, the complexity of human motivation and behaviour is ignored.

Subjective Expected Utility theory

A second and related model is that of Subjective Expected Utility (SEU) theory. This model was also developed in the 1950s (Edwards,1954). It is hypothesised that for any given course of action, an individual will envisage a range of possible outcomes. Each of the possible outcomes is weighted by a subjective probability that the action will lead to that outcome, and the individual will attribute a set of subjective values to each outcome. The sum of these subjective values, or utilities, is said to be the subjective expected utility for that action. Thus, when faced with the need to decide on one of several courses of action, an individual will choose the one with the greatest subjective expected utility. A smoker faced with the decision of whether to stop or continue smoking will follow the path which she or he believes that, on balance, will provide her or him with maximum benefit and minimum cost. For example, a smoker who believes that stopping smoking would greatly improve her/his health and who values physical health more than she/he fears withdrawal symptoms is likely to attempt to stop, whilst a smoker who believes that the psychological benefits to be gained from smoking are very real and who is less convinced by the evidence of increased risk of disease is unlikely to do so. This 'decisional balance' is clearly analogous to the proximal precursors of the Health Belief Model, but includes an element of perceived likelihood of a given action having a given outcome. A further feature of SEU theory which improves its applicability to smoking behaviour is that it is quite compatible with any degree of nicotine dependence. From the point of view of the model, unpleasant or negative subjective values simply contribute to overall subjective expected utility, irrespective of the fact that such outcomes are psychopharmacological in origin. One study which applies SEU theory to cigarette smoking is that of Sutton and Eiser (1984).

Whilst their study was primarily concerned with the effect of fear-arousing communications on smoking behaviour, it showed that a smoker's intention to attempt to stop will depend on:

1. the subjective utility of lung cancer;
2. the perceived reduction in the risk of getting lung cancer following cessation; and
3. the subjective probability of successfully stopping, which they term confidence.

The authors found that the effect of confidence on intention to stop was large: this has important implications for components of the other models discussed below.

Another study which applies SEU theory to smoking behaviour is that of Sutton, Marsh and Matheson (1987). This study was based on a large ($n = 966$) representative sample of smokers drawn from the UK general population. The authors emphasise the importance of confidence in one's ability to stop smoking as part of the model. This is because an attempt to stop smoking may result in success or failure, and confidence in ability to stop smoking is one of the most influential of the array of subjective probabilities considered by the prospective ex-smoker. The results of this study suggest that in any attempt to understand smokers' decisions to stop smoking, prior behaviour must be taken into account: the number of previous attempts was shown to have an effect on intentions that was independent of SEU and confidence. An important finding in this context was that, far from discouraging further attempts, an individual's having made a number of failed attempts seems to strengthen the resolve to stop and was not associated with loss of confidence.

The idea of confidence described by Sutton et al. is clearly comparable with Bandura's (1977) 'self-efficacy' concept. However, the emphasis placed on self-efficacy as a controlling variable in smoking cessation studies (for example, McIntyre, Lichtenstein & Marmelstein, 1983) is done at the expense of motivational variables. It is insufficient to simply believe oneself capable of doing something; it is also necessary to want to do it.

An important shortcoming of SEU theory should be clear, particularly in the context of cigarette smoking. The model does not easily accommodate an element of physical and/or psychological dependence on a psychopharmacologically active substance, such as nicotine. However, as Sutton (1987) points out, the model is concerned with the expectations of the individual, irrespective of their origin. Nevertheless, such reservations are important in situations involving a high degree of psychopharmacological dependence and some authors suggest (Cooper & Croyle, 1984) that perhaps the most integrated model of social behaviours is provided by the Theory of Reasoned Action.

The Theory of Reasoned Action

Two closely related models, the Theory of Reasoned Action (TRA), proposed by Icek Ajzen and Martin Fishbein (1980), and the Theory of Planned Behaviour (Ajzen & Madden, 1986), have been highly influential in health promotion for nearly three decades. In contrast to the shortcomings of the HBM, proponents of these models point out that that they are highly specific, particularly in the way in which their variables are combined. The models also provide an apparently rigorous method for generating relevant beliefs (Mullen, Hersey & Iverson, 1987; Sutton, 1987). The major tenets of these models have either tacitly or explicitly provided a basis for many health promotion interventions. These began with early teaching materials for use in schools (for example, TACADE/HEC, 1984), individual advice (for example, HEC, 1986) and mass media campaigns both in the UK (for example, BBC/HEA, 1990), and the USA (Bauman, 1987), as well as being influential on basic texts on health education theory and practice (for example, Ewles & Simnett, 1985).

Fishbein and Ajzen argue that the immediate determinant of an individual's behaviour is her/his behavioural intention to perform that behaviour (BI). This argument assumes that the behaviour in question is under volitional control, an assumption which is discussed below. It follows therefore that intention should be the best predictor of behaviour. Intention itself is held to be a function of two major determinants, the first of which is concerned with the individual's perception of the positive or negative results of performing the behaviour. This factor is termed the attitude toward the behaviour (AB). The second determinant is concerned with the person's beliefs that important others think she or he should or should not perform that behaviour, and is termed the subjective norm for that behaviour (SN). In general, it is assumed that an individual who has strong intentions is likely to carry out a certain action, and that the strength of that intention in turn will depend on a positive attitude toward the behaviour and the belief that it will meet with approval from other people important to that individual.

The two components are assumed to combine additively to determine behavioural intention thus:

$$BI = w1(AB) + w2(SN)$$

where w1 and w2 are weightings that represent the relative importance of the attitudinal and normative components, which will differ both from individual to individual and from one set of circumstances to another for any given individual.

AB and SN are themselves each held to be determined by two components. AB is said to be a function of the sum of an individual's beliefs that the action in question will have certain given outcomes (for example, 'my smoking will make my baby underweight when it's born'). These beliefs are termed behavioural beliefs. Each behavioural belief is said to be weighted by an outcome evaluation, being an assessment of the degree of perceived desirability/undesirability of the outcome. It is possible, therefore, for an individual to hold a behavioural belief (for example, 'my smoking will make my baby smaller when it's born') which has outcome evaluations that are negative ('low birthweight babies are at more risk') or outcome evaluations that are positive ('a smaller baby would be easier to deliver').

Similarly, SN is held to be a function of two components. The first is whether or not specific referents would approve of the individual performing a given behaviour. These judgements are known as normative beliefs to the action. The second component is composed of a set of weightings which describe how much the individual wishes to comply with each referent's views on their performing that action, and these weights are termed motivations to comply.

The Theory of Planned Behaviour is essentially identical to the TRA, but includes an additional variable known as Perceived Behavioural Control (PBC), which is said to operate directly on behavioural intention.

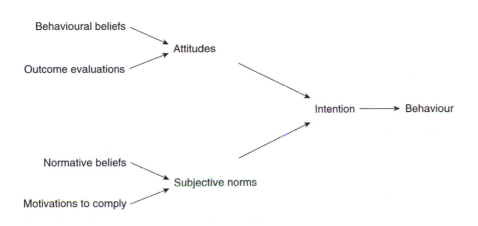

In summary, an individual's intentions, and consequent behaviour, depend on a combination of their beliefs regarding the consequences of the action, and the likely reactions of important others (and, according to the TPB, the degree of control the individual feels they have over that behaviour). In devising health promotion programmes, it is concluded that in order to change an individual's behaviour, it is necessary to change their underlying beliefs. It is this conclusion that has influenced a substantial proportion of health promotion activities for many years. It is the source of repeated attempts to modify people's beliefs as a core component of health promotion programmes.

Reasoned action?

There are many shortcomings to such approaches. Some of these are technical in nature and have been described comprehensively by Sutton (1987). Firstly, it is suggested that the models fail to distinguish between intentions and expectations. Intentions are, it is argued, concerned with one's plans for the future, whilst expectations are simply a measure of perceived likelihood of one's future behaviour (Warshaw & Davis, 1985). Intentions must therefore include expectations, but not vice versa. As a result, a smoker may expect to smoke (or quit) in the future without having formed a plan.

Secondly, a specific concern regarding the Hawthorne effect is raised by Budd and Spencer (1985) and Budd (1987). It is suggested that requiring subjects to complete a questionnaire in the recommended format may lead them to develop attitudes which they did not have in the first place. Thirdly, the models assume that different behavioural beliefs are independent of each other. For example, 'my doctor would like me to stop smoking' is seen as a normative belief whilst 'my stopping smoking would please my doctor' is seen as a behavioural belief. Miniard and Cohen (1981) criticise this aspect of the theory and suggest that because the components are not clearly separated, it leads to 'double-counting' in statistical analyses which make the models appear to have greater predictive ability than they actually possess. Sutton (1989) further points out that even if the two components are conceptually distinct, they are typically correlated, despite such a correlation being reported rarely in published studies.

Further, the simple additive structure of the model does not allow for feedback, either as reciprocal action between the components, or direct action of distal on proximal components (Bentler & Speckart, 1979; Manstead, Proffitt & Smart, 1983; Lucas, 1994).

An additional problem concerns the nature of the weightings w1 and w2 applied to the relative contributions of AB and SN on behavioural intention. According to the model, the values of these weightings vary from individual to individual and from behaviour to behaviour within an individual. If this is the case, both sources of variation clearly must require further psychological interpretation.

There also appear to be inconsistencies between the recommended operationalisations of the model's components (Ajzen & Fishbein, 1980, Appendix A) in that whilst normative belief questions are phrased in terms of the specific behaviour, motivation to comply questions are not, and this despite the emphasis placed by the model on correspondence. Further, Schlegel, Crawford and Sanborn (1977) found that multiplying normative beliefs by motivations to comply actually reduced the model's predictive power. Sutton suggests that normative aspects of behaviour should be regarded simply as perceived rewards and costs, rather than as having any particular status different to other behavioural beliefs. A related criticism is made by Rutter and Bunce (1989). They point out that whilst the model is concerned with individuals' beliefs, respondents are normally asked about belief statements supplied by the experimenter. Their study utilised both the respondents' own belief statements and those supplied by the authors. Whilst respondents' own belief statements produced somewhat stronger predictions for intentions and present behaviour, this was not the case for subsequent behaviour measured at 8 weeks follow-up. Similarly, Burnkrant and Page (1988) suggest that the normative belief/motivation to comply component is multidimensional, rather than a single construct, and that such multidimensional constructs are differentially predictive of SN.

A further limitation to the theories lies in their failure to incorporate any measure of past behaviour. Clearly, long-established behaviours are likely to induce a certain degree of inertia, particularly if an habitual component or psychopharmacological dependence may be involved. This may in turn result in correlation values between the model's components and behaviour being misleadingly large. Certainly, some studies have found that not only does past behaviour have a substantial effect on current intention and future behaviour (Bentler & Speckart, 1979; Lucas, 1994), but also that intention, whilst itself a significant predictor of future drug use, increased prediction over and above that by previous substance use only minimally. Further, this finding is not confined to studies which involve dependence-forming substances. Charng, Piliavin and Callero (1988) found that including a measure of habit significantly improved prediction of intention and behaviour in a study of blood donation. However, Chassin et al.'s (1984) study of smoking behaviour in adolescents analysed their results for never-smokers, experimental smokers and regular smokers separately, thus controlling for previous behaviour. This study showed that, at least in terms of the relationship between AB and BI, no effect from previous behaviour appeared to be operating. Similar findings emerge from Sherman et al.'s (1982) study of smoking behaviour.

Other limitations exist in relation to the TRA and TPB, mainly concerned with the practicalities of operationalisation. Firstly, applications of these theories typically employ questionnaires using a semantic differential format. In practice, phrasing some of the outcomes of 'risky' behaviours in the recommended manner results in somewhat peculiar questions; for example, 'Would your getting lung cancer be good/bad?' This is inevitable given that applications in health promotion often require respondents to evaluate potentially serious, or even fatal outcomes.

Secondly, and more importantly, previous studies have shown that outcome evaluations usually contribute little to the predictive power of the model; the variation in such outcome evaluations is generally very small in such applications and thus does not contribute meaningfully to prediction.

Thirdly, any application of the model which includes an adequately comprehensive range of behavioural beliefs necessitates constructing a questionnaire of considerable length. While this is generally not an issue with the samples employed in many published studies (often of university students), application to a more general population can be problematic (Lucas, 1994). Debate continues as to precisely how the models should best be operationalised.

The Transtheoretical ('Stages of Change') Model

A different approach to explaining health-related behaviour is taken by Prochaska and DiClemente (1983). Their work is based on a model developed in the psychotherapy literature (Prochaska, 1979; Prochaska & DiClemente, 1982a) and from studies of self-change (Prochaska & DiClemente, 1982b). The model has been particularly widely applied to attempts to stop people smoking, and is therefore described here in such terms. In this model, Prochaska and DiClemente propose five 'stages of change': pre-contemplation, contemplation, action, maintenance and relapse. Among cigarette smokers they report that quitters used the fewest processes of change during pre-contemplation, emphasised consciousness-raising during the contemplation stage, emphasised self re-evaluation in both contemplation and action stages, emphasised self-liberation, a helping relationship and reinforcement management during the action stage and used counterconditioning and stimulus control the most in both action and maintenance stages.

Limitations of the Transtheoretical Model

Recently several authors have noted limitations to this model. Firstly, it has been suggested that there is little empirical evidence for the existence of the distinct stages the model proposes, let alone that they exist in the circular order suggested by Prochaska and DiClemente.

An illustration of this criticism may be seen in relation to smoking behaviour. In this domain, the model's stages are often defined as follows:

- Pre-contemplation: one who is not contemplating quitting in the next six months
- Preparation: one who is planning to quit in the next 30 days and who has made at least one attempt lasting one day or more in the last 12 months
- Contemplation: everybody else.

Even these basic algorithms present problems. Firstly, the classification is arbitrary: why not three months and seven days instead of six months and thirty days? Secondly, the stage construct is, in Fishbein's terminology, a composite of intention and behaviour. More seriously, Sutton (1996) has pointed out that according to the model, a smoker cannot be in the preparation stage unless they have made a recent quit attempt. It follows that the first time they tried to quit, they must have done so without being in the preparation stage. A smoker can thus never be 'prepared' for his/her first quit attempt. Similarly, Stockwell (1996) asks:

> how reliably different are smokers who are 'contemplating quitting smoking in the next six months' versus those who are not? What does it mean to be contemplating such a thing? Does one have to be contemplating this now, five minutes ago, sometime today or in the past week? Surely every smoker these days contemplates quitting at regular intervals? (p. 1283)

A more detailed criticism of the stages of change model in predicting smoking cessation is provided by Farkas et al. (1996). They found that when stage of change was used as a stand-alone predictor, smokers in 'preparation' at baseline were more likely than those in 'pre-contemplation' to be abstinent at follow-up. However, when stage membership was combined with measures of pharmacological addiction, the former no longer predicted cessation. Moreover, occasional versus daily smoking, number of cigarettes smoked and lifetime number of quits discriminated abstinence much better at follow-up than did stages of change; the overall prediction by stage of change model yielded 55% whilst overall prediction by the addition model yielded nearly 70%. Farkas and his colleagues conclude that:

> our results question the utility of the stages of change construct as a predictor of smoking cessation. Although smokers in the preparation stage at baseline showed higher rates of cessation one to two years later, we observed no difference in follow-up cessation rates between those in the contemplation stage and those in the pre-contemplation stage at baseline. Furthermore, stage of change was not an independent predictor when used in the multivariate analysis with other predictors. (p. 1277)

Other researchers are even more explicit in their criticism. For example, Pierce et al. (1996) found no significant difference in quitting history by stage of change in a longitudinal study of over 2000 smokers. They conclude:

> While we agree that the stage of change model has had considerable historical importance in getting clinicians to accept behaviour change as a process, this does not mean that it has successfully ousted earlier paradigms in health promotion. Before we put any theory on such a

pedestal we should carefully scrutinise its performance compared with the previously accepted theories. This is particularly so for a model that has been accused of achieving prominence with a relative absence of scientific support for its validity. (p. 1291)

It is certainly true that this model has, as Pierce suggests, been 'put on a pedestal'. By October 1997, a UK training programme called Helping People Change had over 500 trainers throughout England (HEA, 1997). These trainers taught a course with a 12 hour core, plus several additional four-hour-modules, based on Prochaska and DiClemente's stages of change model. The main target audience for this training was primary care professionals and allied workers. Well over 4500 practitioners were trained by 1997.

Of course health promotion programmes must be underpinned by theory and be capable of rigorous objective analysis. At the same time, the inadequacy of strategies based solely on theory has been repeatedly illustrated by the failure of many intervention programmes to date.

The question remains, whether it is possible to explain health-related behaviour more extensivelly. For a start, we can look at the phenomenon we are interested in (in this case, people). Real people are much more complex than many social psychological models would have us believe. As an example, we offer adolescent smoking, an area rightly of concern to health promoters. What follows are conclusions from a study we conducted for the UK Department of Health (Lloyd & Lucas, 1997). We investigated many aspects of adolescent cigarette smoking, including measuring components of some of the models described above, but we also investigated a range of much broader factors than beliefs and intentions. While small amounts of variance in smoking behaviour were predicted by attitudes, subjective norms and all the other familiar components, much more was predicted by quite different factors.

Although disappointing to those looking for a 'quick fix' to prevent teenagers from smoking, it must be acknowledged that many of these factors are difficult to influence by conventional, mass-media or classroom interventions. They are generally factors over which adolescents have little or no control (for example, family breakdown and divorce), or a result of influences beyond the personal or familial (for example, the lack of a coherent sense of community or communal identity). For example, there is a complex relationship between age, gender and physical maturity which has a powerful effect on smoking uptake among adolescent girls. This relationship is shown in Figure 5.1.

Here, it can be seen that the relationship between sexual maturity and smoking among boys is a fairly straightforward one. At any given age, boys who have reached puberty are more likely to smoke than are boys of the same age who have not yet reached puberty. However, for girls, the relationship is more complex. Like boys, post-pubescent girls up to the age

Figure 5.1   Smoothed estimates of smoking prevalence by gender, age and physical maturity

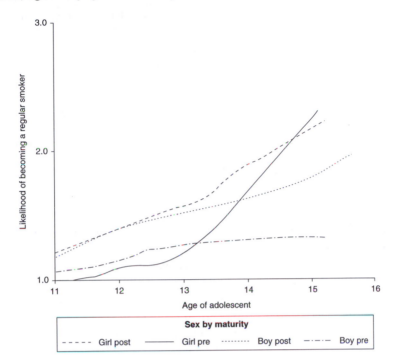

Source: Lloyd & Lucas, 1998

of 13–14 years are more likely to smoke than are pre-pubescent girls of the same age. But as they approach 14 years of age, there is a sharp inflexion in the curve: at 15, pre-pubescent girls are equally likely to smoke as are their more mature contemporaries, and by just over 15 they become *more* likely to be smokers. This relationship is exemplified further in Table 5.1. This shows the results of a discriminant function analysis using a model developed from insights gained from a LOWESS plot. A variable was created to take account of the influence upon girls' smoking behaviour of the interaction of age and maturity. This variable, along with age, gender, maturity, and an age by gender interaction served as discriminators.

The success of the multiple discriminant analysis is assessed by its ability to identify group membership – 64% of pupils who had never smoked could be successfully predicted. This is unsurprising since smoking is relatively rare among the youngest groups in the study (11 years). *However, 71% of regular smokers aged 11–16 can be predicted on the basis of age, gender and sexual maturity* **alone**.

This level of prediction is far greater than that generally achieved by the most sophisticated applications of social cognition models. *But more importantly, smoking is predicted by* **immutable** *variables: gender, age and*

Table 5.1   Discriminant function classification of smoking group membership

Actual group	No. of cases	Predicted group membership		
		1	2	3
Never (1)	1999	1275	303	421
	%	**64**	15	21
Occasional (2)	1025	408	200	417
	%	40	**20**	41
Regular (3)	371	52	57	262
	%	14	15	**71**

All of these variables were significant at the $p < .001$ level (F statistics with $df = 3392,2$).

sexual maturity. Such characteristics cannot be manipulated by simple anti-smoking health promotion interventions.

A further clear finding from our study was that adolescents living with both parents are less likely to smoke, or to take up smoking during the course of the school year, than are those living in single-parent families, or stepfamilies. This finding remained *after controlling for parental smoking behaviour* (Lloyd & Lucas, 1998). These results are shown in Table 5.2 below.

Ours is only one of a number of studies from around the world which consistently report this observation. For example, Green et al. (1990) in Scotland showed that while the children of single mothers were more likely to smoke, there was no evidence that they did so *because* their mothers smoked; children of single mothers were actually less likely to be smokers than were the children of mothers who lived with a new partner rather than the child's father. In Finland, Isohanni et al. (1991) found that children from 'non-standard' families were significantly more likely to smoke than were

Table 5.2   Family structure and smoking behaviour

Family structure	% Never smokers	% Occasional smokers	% Regular smokers	N
Both parents	**60.9**	29.6	**9.5**	2616
Mother and stepfather	42.7	39.3	16.1	321
Mother only	48.5	39.9	11.6	474
Father and stepmother	53.3	30.0	16.7	30
Father only	48.4	31.3	20.3	64
Neither parent	**41.7**	29.2	**29.2**	24

Source: Lloyd & Lucas, 1998

those raised by both biological parents. More specifically, Bailey et al. (1993) found smoking among Australian teenagers to be *independently* linked to familial characteristics such as family disunion. Similarly, in the USA, Doherty and Allen (1994) found poorer family functioning, and lower family cohesion, to be *independently* predictive of adolescent smoking.

Findings such as these should not produce too much surprise. Is it so unexpected that adolescents who feel secure and are happier with their sense of identity have fewer difficulties? Is it really so unlikely that children who are brought up by both biological parents in a supportive and caring environment are less likely to exhibit health-related problem behaviours than those who live in discord or those who have to adjust to a new (or a succession of) parent-figures?

Why then are the models considered in this chapter so attractive to health professionals? At least seven reasons may be adduced:

- The models are relatively easy to understand
- They provide an explanation as to why interventions don't always work
- They provide a reason why some clients don't want to change
- They provide more readily achievable goals: not just 'all or nothing'
- They are applicable (simultaneously) to a wide range of behaviours
- They locate a practitioner's input into the context of the client's experience
- Historically, paradigm shifts are always exciting.

Decades of failure to influence health behaviour substantially suggest that there are at least two additional considerations which are not included in any of these models. Firstly, decision-making processes are not always rational. Second and more importantly, individual decision-making is not the sole determinant of human behaviour.

The complexity of the decision-making process in the adoption of health-related behaviours need not be framed in such mechanistic and mutually exclusive terms. The motivation of ordinary people is much more complex than social cognition and other models would have us believe. Moreover, much health promotion activity has been predicated on somewhat simplistic interpretations of influential theories, in which an individual's decisions are interpreted as logical and straightforward. Motivation for engaging in a given behaviour is not simply the polar opposite of motivation for avoiding that behaviour. Even within the constraints of such paradigms, motivations for and against engagement have been shown to be commonly very *different* entities (Lucas, 1994), each carrying with them constellations of associated outcomes which are embedded in an individual's social world, *over aspects of which many people have little or no direct personal influence.*

However, in this volume we are more concerned with *human* perspectives. Our most fundamental criticism of these approaches concerns their philosophy and appropriateness in relation to human behaviours. Do people really weigh up the benefits and costs of a particular action in such a precise, methodical and analytical way? Do people really go through discrete, mutually exclusive 'stages' of behaviour? As Roberts, Towell and Golding (2001) observe:

> if we take the observation that most people simply don't perceive themselves to be at risk of ill-health (this is certainly true for young people smoking and drinking to excess as well as engaging in unplanned and unprotected sexual behaviour), then logically one might consider means to alter perceived susceptibility. However, although when questioned respondents may acknowledge the potentially severe consequences of their action (such as lung cancer, liver damage or HIV infection), the long delay between the action and its potentially adverse consequences constitutes a strong barrier to effective learning. (p. 80)

We would argue that the reason why such models predict behaviour poorly is the same reason that health promotion strategies based on them have, at least to date, been disappointing in terms of changing people's behaviour. The key question, Roberts and colleagues propose, is whether these models lead to viable effective strategies or the likelihood of developing them.

The attempt to provide a 'scientific' basis for health promotion interventions (at least partly driven by medical paradigms) has resulted in an approach which, in our view, is reductionist to an extent which ignores the complexity of whole human beings. The meticulous study of the social-psychological trees has blinded health promoters to the human wood. To attempt to explain human behaviour solely on the basis of selected participants' responses to carefully crafted questionnaire items is, in our view, analogous to attempting to describe symphonic music solely in terms of a timed series of sound frequencies. People (not 'subjects', 'clients', 'patients' or even 'participants') are much more than collections of behavioural beliefs, subjective norms and intentions. It is these other qualities which are likely to prove impossible to reduce to sets of data points while retaining their complexity and integrity.

Roberts et al. (2001: 80) are very pessimistic in their view of social cognition (and related) models in planning health promotion programmes. In relation to the TRA and TPB, they assert that 'the manner in which [these models] describe the processes governing behaviour must be regarded as fundamentally misleading'. As reasons, they point firstly to their linear nature, and their lack of consideration of the habitual nature of many of the behaviours to which they are applied, suggesting that:

> to capture complex context dependent behaviour within a linear individual centred framework is doomed to failure ... the choices people

make cannot be extricated from the choices that others make, nor from the power relations between them, nor the wider social milieu which dictates the availability of choice and sets limits to personal efficacy and control. (p. 80)

There is some evidence to support such a view. A recent meta-analytic review of the Theory of Planned Behaviour reports that while 39% of intention can be predicted from the model's proximal components, overall the model can only account for 27% of variance in behaviour. Moreover, the TPB accounted for 11% more variance in self-reported behaviour than in studies which employed objective or observed measures of behaviour (Armitage & Conner, 2001). Even Icek Ajzen (1998), writing of applications of such models to health psychology, notes that 'few profound insights have as yet resulted from their application, with the possible exception of the recognition that self-regulation, and especially self-efficacy, plays a major role in all aspects of health, illness and recovery' (p. 735).

Yet despite these difficulties, we believe that such approaches should not be ignored. Social cognition models have made a significant contribution to health psychology. It may be, as Roberts et al. (2001) suggest, that more sophisticated modelling techniques will advance their utility further. More recent work has pointed to the need to incorporate other components into these models which may improve their predictive ability, including perceived need (Paisley & Sparks, 1998), post-decisional cognitive processes (Abraham et al., 1999), anticipated regret (Abraham & Sheeran, 2003b) and goal theories (Abraham & Sheeran, 2003a), extraversion and self-esteem (Wilkinson & Abraham, 2004).

Our view is that discussion of the merits of these models will continue long after the writing of this volume. We would certainly concur with Ajzen when he suggests that the advantage of models such as the Theory of Planned Behaviour lies in their applicability across behavioural domains, and that their major utility 'has been to organise and communicate knowledge about health-related behaviour' (Ajzen, 1998: 735).

From the viewpoint of planning practical health promotion activities, we suggest that social cognition models do offer some explanations for people's behaviour, but incomplete ones. In order to understand why people do what they do, we need to look more at whole people, not just sets of attitudes, beliefs and intentions. Whole people also have emotions, hopes, fears, friends, families, life histories and cultures. These things may be more difficult to measure reliably with scales, and may be less amenable to complex and elegant statistical analyses. They are also more difficult to attempt to influence in health promotion schemes. But if we adopt such a view, we believe that those programmes may be more realistic and successful.

SIX Risky behaviour?
Judging the odds

The policy of being too cautious is the greatest risk of all.

Jawaharlal Nehru

And the trouble is, if you don't risk anything, you risk even more.

Erica Jong

On a visit to Portugal the first author and a public health colleague visited a new social centre. The foyer was painted a wonderfully peaceful shade of blue that drew the eye repeatedly. Here, older people have lunch, talk, play dominoes and are generally sociable. However, there is a radical difference between this facility and those in the UK: these facilities are shared with pre-school children. An old man makes paper aeroplanes for the children to throw across the lawn; an elderly lady teaches a little girl a nursery rhyme. When we express surprise, our guide (a social worker) tells us that all such facilities in Lisbon usually mix older people and young children under the same roof. She is astonished to learn that we do not do so in the UK. 'Why do you put your old people into ghettos?' she asks. 'What have they done wrong? The children need to be looked after because their parents work. The old people like to see young people. This way, both are happy.' The simple logic of her question was very difficult to answer.

Back home, we shared this experience with professional colleagues. The reactions were depressingly predictable: 'What about the risks of sexual abuse?' … 'Just think of the increased risk of cross-infection.'

Privately, we concluded that these are rationalisations for a lack of vision rather than justifiable concerns, and illustrate cultural differences in the construction of groups in society.

Introduction

In this chapter we consider some of the more influential models and ideologies that have been developed to describe health promotion as an emergent discipline. A large volume of literature has been amassed in which various models have been described, compared and contrasted, and this process of reflective self-examination has been roughly continuous throughout the ontology of health promotion as a profession. This exercise has been extensively covered elsewhere, even becoming the major focus of an important volume (Downie, Tannahill & Tannahill, 1996). Our intention here is not to repeat such an analysis but merely to outline the major features of this development in order to set the main focus of this chapter: the degree to which these models have influenced health promotion activity. Cigarette smoking and attempts to persuade smokers to quit are used as illustrative examples. Finally, proposals for alternative approaches are suggested.

Few occupational groups have been afflicted with a greater number and diversity of ideological models in such a short space of time as those people said to be 'working in health promotion'. We use this generic phrase because successive changes in outlook, political constraints and fashion are clearly illustrated by the rapid evolution of job titles of such individuals. In the early-to-mid 1980s, most people in the UK working in this field were generally known as 'Health *Education* Officers' of various grades and levels of seniority. By the mid-to-late 1980s, such workers (to a large extent the same individuals) were very insistent that they now be known as 'Health *Promotion* Officers' in order to reflect the broader remit that changes in contemporary ideologies permitted their job descriptions to include. This change was concurrent with an increasingly common view that a postgraduate qualification, then only available from a handful of polytechnics, was the *sine qua non* of a successful applicant for such a position. Shortly after this time, the title 'Officer' was considered to sound far too authoritarian and was therefore seamlessly transmuted to 'Adviser' and occasionally (and especially, contemporary cynics commented, in the most politically-correct departments) to 'Facilitator'.

By contrast to this movement toward greater liberalness, it is perhaps ironic that during this same period, the flagship health promotion organisation for England and Wales changed its title from the Health Education *Council* to the Health Education *Authority*. This change was accompanied by a tightening of its corporate remit, including removal of its professional development and some of its research and development functions. In 2000 this long-suffering and (within the field) often-maligned organisation was disbanded only to re-emerge as the Health Development Agency (HDA). Although precisely how health is to be 'developed' remains to be demonstrated, some workers now describe themselves as 'working in health development'. This uncertainty is not particularly alleviated by the HDA's somewhat impenetrable description of its own activities:

> The HDA focuses on the development of the public health workforce through a variety of means in order to ensure the delivery of health improvement. ... Evidence is channelled into policymaking through direct policy comment and facilitation and support of the implementation of public health policy. ... The translation of evidence into improved practice is achieved through a variety of means including evidence based guidance, supporting the delivery of health improvement through public health workforce planning, the development of tools of change such as learning from practice, the appropriate use of standard setting processes and the facilitation and support of partnerships. The range of methods are also applied within settings with young people and in the workplace. (HDA, 2004)

Yet throughout this period, the day-to-day activities carried out by most people working in health promotion changed far less than their appellations might have suggested. Despite notable exceptions involving the major government funding of socially-orientated projects such as Surestart, the focus of *most* health promotion activity remains centred around reducing the incidence of coronary heart disease and certain cancers, drug misuse and HIV infection rates, mainly by attempting to alter health-related behaviours.

Health education

Nearly a quarter of a century ago, Draper and colleagues (1980) identified what they saw as three types of health education: firstly, that concerned with the body and how to look after it; secondly, that which provides information about access to health services; and thirdly, education about policies, structures and processes in the environment which may be detrimental to health. Each of Draper's 'types' has been criticised, both by academics and by health promotion field workers. The first type may lead to what became known as 'victim-blaming' in which failure to conform to a set of prescribed 'healthy' behaviours results in various kinds of ill health, the key feature being that such outcomes would be the individual's own fault. Similarly, it has been widely held that Draper's second 'type' is flawed because of its reliance on the lead of experts and allegiance to medical models, with no room for individual choice or responsibility;

these are limitations which may also be argued to apply to Draper's third 'type' of health education. Clearly, Draper's own medical background and, arguably, the original vehicle chosen to discuss his typology (the *British Medical Journal*), were influences on this early work. Nevertheless, and despite such criticisms, Downie et al. (1996) point out that the first of Draper's types – giving people information about their own bodies and their upkeep, a concern which became widely known throughout the 1980s as 'body maintenance' – is an essential starting point, and is one which continues to rightly attract substantial sums of funding to this day.

It was at this time that much academic activity focused around linking individual health-related behaviour and social psychological theory (some limitations of which are discussed in detail in Chapter 5). Social psychologists strove to improve the link between knowledge, as provided by Draper's first 'type', and the desired behavioural changes which might reduce an individual's risk of becoming ill. While this kind of academic research and health promotion activity continues unabated, we would argue that evidence of success in modifying behaviour by such means has proved at best limited (for example, in the case of promoting safer sex) and at worst absent (for example, in the case of preventing teenage smoking). More importantly, such an approach still regards health promotion as essentially being about reducing the risk of certain diseases.

One social-psychological construct which has received much attention from health promoters is that of locus of control, which may be seen as a particular dimension of attribution theory (Heider, 1944; 1958). Attribution theory suggests that people desire to view their worlds as controllable and predictable, and to do this it is necessary to make attributions about cause and effect in their everyday lives. Such ideas were developed by Herzlich (1973). In an interview study of 80 subjects, Herzlich noted that 'health' was regarded as something 'internal' to an individual, while 'illness' was regarded as something 'external', something which came in from the outside world. Such sets of attributions have been shown to influence patients' choice of treatment modalities in diabetes (Bradley, 1985), and attendance at blood pressure screening clinics (King, 1982). What has become known as health locus of control (Wallston & Wallston, 1982) has provided measures of whether individuals believe their health status to be controlled by themselves (internal health locus of control) or by external agencies over which they have no control, or by 'fate' (external health locus of control).

Wallston and Wallston (1982) developed this concept into a specifically health-orientated scale of locus of control. This work subsequently generated a large volume of research across many health-related behaviours, gave birth to a number of specialised locus of control scales, and has been widely embraced by health promotion workers for two reasons. Firstly, the general notion is that an individual's health locus of control can help explain health-related behaviour. For example, a smoker whose health locus of control is primarily external may be more likely to believe that his/her health is mainly determined by the results of fate, chance or random hazards in everyday life and may thus be less likely to see benefits in stopping smoking, while smoking may be an activity less likely to be found among more 'internal' individuals who believe their health to be primarily determined by personal behaviour.

Secondly, it follows that if it were possible to somehow shift an individual's health locus of control from an external to a more internal state, then that individual could be predicted to change their behaviour away from pathogenic activities such as smoking, excessive drinking and sedentary living towards more healthy alternatives. One obvious appeal of such a concept to health promoters and governments alike is that it is simultaneously consistent with liberal notions of empowerment and with more conservative ideals of personal responsibility.

However, the seductiveness of this concept is not without difficulties, both theoretical and practical. Firstly, people are not consistently internal or external in their attributions regarding health. For example, one's risk of lung cancer may be attributed internally (among non-smokers at least) while one's risk of other cancers may easily be construed as 'fate', 'genetic' or even 'luck'. Secondly, the decision to use medical services may be both internal and external: seeking medical advice may be internal in that it involves taking control, but is external in that it puts responsibility into the hands of experts or 'powerful others'.

Secondly, the concept of health locus of control suffers the same limitations of many other social-psychological constructs in terms of their practical utility to health promotion programmes. To be useful, it is necessary to be able to *change* locus of control (assuming it is a simple, constant feature of an individual) by the limited means available to health promoters. Like many such concepts, the theory helps identify individuals towards whom interventions may be directed, but offers little guidance about what the content of such interventions might be.

Health promotion

Since Draper's early typology, an increasing number of more sophisticated models have been proposed, which have driven the change from discussions of health education to those of health promotion. Tannahill (1985) proposed what has arguably been one of the most quoted and influential models of health promotion. Tannahill sees health promotion as a range of activities which can be visualised as three overlapping circles, much in the manner of a Venn diagram. These three circles respectively represent health education, disease prevention and health protection. Areas where these circles overlap are seen to represent composite activities: for example, the overlap of prevention and education represents 'educational efforts to influence lifestyle in the interests of preventing ill-health, as well as efforts to encourage the uptake of preventive services' (Tannahill, 1985, cited in Downie et al., 1996: 59). Similarly, the area where the circles of prevention and health protection overlap is described as 'preventive health protection', for example in the fluoridation of drinking water to help prevent dental caries. From our perspective, while such models have demonstrably added to the range of activities that distinguish health promotion from health education, they are of themselves at times somewhat pedantic classifications and not particularly helpful in practice. For example, are 'educational' (as opposed to commercial) efforts to influence lifestyle likely to be aimed at anything other than preventing ill health? Similarly, such terms occasionally appear to be oxymoronic ('preventive health protection measures'). The practical usefulness of such terms is sometimes less than clear.

Moreover, activities which may be described as 'preventive health protection' may not be as justified as well-meaning instigators believe them to be. For example, Marshall (2000) triggered a spirited debate by suggesting the introduction of what he describes as a 'fiscal food policy'. Such a policy would, he argued, prevent between 900 and 1000 premature deaths a year in the UK. At the time of writing, most food sold in Britain is exempt from value added tax (VAT). Because diet determines blood cholesterol concentrations, Marshall argues, and blood cholesterol concentrations determine the prevalence of ischaemic heart disease, then reducing the amount of dietary cholesterol consumed by the British public will inevitably reduce the prevalence of CHD. As public levels of purchasing of most commodities is determined by price, Marshall reasons, increasing the cost of fatty foods at the checkout should reduce sales and thus consumption of these products among the poor, who as a result will inevitably lead healthier, longer lives. Moreover, he continues, the increased tax revenue so raised could be used to compensate the NHS (and society in general) for the costs resulting from illnesses that those who persist in purchasing such foods bring upon themselves.

To support his argument, Marshall (an epidemiologist) cites the impressive 'Keyes Equation' (Keyes et al., 1965; Clarke et al., 1997; Tang et al., 1998) by which a potential change in serum cholesterol may be calculated for a given change in the proportion of saturated fats consumed. By the use of this equation, Marshall notes that a fall of 0.6 mmol/l in blood cholesterol concentrations should bring about a 25–30% fall in the incidence of ischaemic heart disease within five years (Holme, 1990; Law et al., 1994), and concludes that such estimates are conservative.

However, is such an apparently simple measure an answer to the problems of obesity and coronary heart disease which are so prevalent in contemporary Britain? After all, repeated increases in the cost of cigarettes have long been advocated (and employed) in attempts to reduce tobacco consumption, and the inverse relationship between the real price of tobacco and consumption is well-established. Nevertheless, smoking rates have remained approximately constant for some years, particularly among the least well-off, and rates have actually increased sharply in some groups, irrespective of increases in price. On the contrary, among teenage girls there is clear evidence that even at higher prices, cigarettes provide what is considered to be an 'affordable accessory' to assist the construction of a desired image [identity] (Lloyd & Lucas, 1998).

However, other workers suggest that Marshall's approach is simplistic and naïve for other reasons. Kennedy and Offutt (2000) (of the US Department of Agriculture) point out a number of flaws in Marshall's proposals which are applicable to Draper's notion of 'preventive health protection' more generally. Firstly, biological problems exist in relation to Marshall's proposal. The way in which an individual (as opposed to a sample mean or population overall) responds to changes in saturated fat intake is determined genetically. For many people, the net response of serum low density and low density lipoprotein cholesterol to reducing dietary cholesterol is, in reality, quite limited (Dreon et al., 1994). A study which illustrates the limitations of this relationship is that of DISC (1995). In this study, children aged 8–10 years who were at high risk were put on a diet containing only 10% of total calories as saturated fat for a period of up to three years. This major change in diet resulted in only a modest effect on their serum cholesterol at the end of the experimental period. Moreover, Kennedy et al. (1999) have shown that the generally-accepted notion that there are sizeable differences in the diets of the rich and poor is now becoming less accurate than was the case previously, at least in the USA; this is because of the increased tendency of both rich and poor to eat away from home. Marshall (2000) concedes that the degree to which increases in cost might actually result in decreases in purchases of high-fat foods (known as 'price elasticity') is uncertain. In any case, empirical evidence from the USA shows that price elasticities are generally much smaller than Marshall assumes, which means that increases in VAT would actually result in far smaller reductions in consumption than he predicts. Taken together, these findings make it seem unlikely that any changes that might realistically be expected to be produced by 'fiscal food policies' would significantly reduce levels of CHD.

Risk as rational

Yet the real concern from our perspective is not solely the unsteady science and (at best) controversial assumptions on which Marshall's proposals are founded. Firstly, there is the criticism of many 'educational' approaches to changing behaviour that we make repeatedly in this book: generally, the risks and advantages of many behavioural changes which seem so obvious and straightforward when applied to populations are more complex at the individual level. Becker (1993) somewhat pointedly cites the findings of Taylor et al. (1987) which put this distinction into context. Taylor and colleagues constructed a model in which they calculated how much increased life expectancy could be predicted to result from a mass dietary cholesterol reduction programme. On average, individuals aged 20–60 who were considered to be at low risk in terms of smoking behaviour, blood pressure and HDLP levels would be able to look forward to an extra 3 days to 3 months of life as a result of reducing their dietary cholesterol, while individuals assessed as high risk (by the same criteria) stood to gain between 18 days and 12 months. Becker notes the understatement in Taylor et al.'s conclusion that 'although there are undoubtedly persons who would choose to participate in a lifelong regimen of dietary change to achieve results of this magnitude, we suspect that some might not' (p. 2).

The issue of confusing risks found in analyses of populations with those for the individual is eloquently (and amusingly) expressed in analogy form by the anthropologist Charlie Davison, who made a study of CHD prevention in Wales (Davison, Davey & Smith Frankel, 1992). Davison likens attempts at the mass reduction of dietary cholesterol to a story in which a lecturer has to get a group of several hundred students onto a train to embark on a journey, in the knowledge that if he succeeds, then one of their lives will be saved. The only problem is that the lecturer does not know which student is the one actually at risk. Undeterred, he goads, threatens and coerces some of them onto the train, knowing that for all but one of them, the journey will have been completely unnecessary. Unsurprisingly, a few of them object but begrudgingly comply, and many more refuse to get on board altogether.

More pertinent still is the implication that it is the business of government to interfere with people's choices when minor risk reductions which might be achieved for a few individuals are forcibly applied to entire populations, with the whole exercise aggrandized with notions of 'fiscal policy' which imply some form of patronising philanthropy.

Citing risks may be a less useful part of the health promoter's repertoire than is generally imagined. We would argue that employing notions of risk which axiomatically assume that everyone is motivated to reduce it to a minimum is both naïve and simplistic. First, different risks mean different things to different people. For example, some individuals take part in sports (such as rock-climbing and hang-gliding) which carry considerable risks; others would never even contemplate participation in such activities because of the dangers involved. Yet for those who do participate, *the risk is actually the point*: it is the excitement during, and sense of achievement after, taking part in high-risk sports in which their very appeal lies. Such 'pleasure-through-danger' has always been a part of human nature throughout history and across all cultures.

Second, which risks are deemed acceptable and which risks are deemed unacceptable is culturally mediated. From a Western health promotion perspective, any activity which increases the risk of physical illness is discouraged, and any activity which reduces such risk is encouraged. Yet these distinctions come with values attached. For example, serious facial and spinal injuries regularly occur in contact sports such as rugby; lower limb injuries are extremely common in running; premature arthritic changes are frequently found in the joints of gymnasts and dancers. Nevertheless, these three activities are generally viewed as courageous, athletic and artistic respectively. Thus athletes and sportspeople are seen as choosing 'healthy activities' which have (generally underplayed) risks and smokers and drinkers (who may simply see themselves as indulging in pleasurable accessories to relaxation) are judged feckless and irresponsible. In the last few decades this selectivity has resulted in suggestions, from both physicians and politicians, to refuse NHS treatment to smokers who develop smoking-related illnesses, while few have suggested that hospitals should turn away spinally-injured rugby players. The tension between health promoters' and public explanations of risky behaviours is expressed eloquently by Roberts et al. (2001) in relation to alcohol use:

> Social learning theories suggest that poor coping resources, the presence of cues to drink and the belief that alcohol will have a positive outcome contribute to excessive drinking. In contrast, the most commonly stated reasons for using alcohol amongst 'normal' drinkers include the relief of tension or anxiety, improving social competence and *producing drunkenness* [our italics]. Building links between these two accounts is necessary in order to develop a viable developmental theory of problem drinking. (p. 108)

Thus it seems that academics and professionals define the reasons people use alcohol in terms of deviancy and misguided belief, while (when asked) drinkers report their reasons for using alcohol to be as an adjunct to normal social life, including pleasurable intoxication for its own sake. The contrast between these two perspectives (and the manner by which data about them are produced) is a theme which runs throughout the present volume.

Third, a number of authors have noted that relative risks are difficult to explain meaningfully to a mass audience. Recent fears over the risk of Bovine Spongiform Encephalopathy (BSE) being passed to humans resulted in a huge reduction in beef sales in the UK, while smoking rates continued to rise among teenagers. The risks of BSE transmission are orders of magnitude lower than the risks of acquiring smoking-related diseases through tobacco use, but the health-related behaviour of much of the British public changed in the direction opposite to that consistent with known risk.

Finally, for many people, personal development is actually dependent on being *less* concerned solely with personal welfare and valetudinarianism. Such a view is a feature of a wide range of religious, spiritual and philosophical beliefs and is explored further below.

The role of social-psychological models

It is thus helpful at this stage to consider precisely what the purpose of social-psychological models might be, and in what ways they can influence priority setting. What has been the utility of the many and various models which crowd the health promotion literature, and of which an understanding represents a substantial portion of the syllabus in many health promotion courses? Tones and Tilford (2001) cite Luck and Luckman's (1974) definition of a model as being:

> a representation of the significant features of the problem under study ... [which is] ... a faithful representation of the problem; ... [and] a powerful tool for examining a wide range of alternative courses of action. (p. 29)

However, when considering the range of sometimes conflicting and often orthogonal models applied to health promotion, such a definition may be considered a little optimistic. Tones and Tilford's (2001) own summary of what a model should be is perhaps a more accurate and useful one:

> a model should provide a simplified representation of some aspect of reality that ... incorporates all of the key elements needed to provide an account of the subject under review. (p. 29)

If the use of models to describe health promotion activity in areas as relatively straightforward as the prevention of CHD and dental disease lack the simplicity that Tones and Tilford rightly favour, then the application of such concepts to more complex activities such as mental health promotion is even more daunting. In a comprehensive and important work on this area of work, Tudor (1996) presents an interesting account of how mental health professionals have attempted to extend or adapt existing models to their fields. For example, Verrall (1990) has suggested an adaptation of Tannahill's (1985) model in which his 'health education' circle represents enhancing well-being, and Tannahill's 'prevention' circle includes services such as counselling and crisis intervention schemes. In his book, Tudor initially presents a complex discourse on the grounding of mental health promotion in sociological theory, but notes that different aspects of mental health fit more readily into different paradigms. However, Tudor then goes on to identify 'from the literature and from practice' what he considers to be 'elements of mental health for mental health promotion, presented as elements for development among individuals' (p. 63). It is this shift which makes Tudor's contribution particularly valuable, as he continues to relate his 'elements of mental health promotion' in policy and practice. It is this grasp of the essentials of an aspect of health and a pragmatic approach to their nurturance that is, in our view, key to the development of more effective health promotion strategies.

The notion of it being the responsibility of individuals to optimise their health by the avoidance of known risk factors depends on the first question asked in many rudimentary health promotion texts: what do we consider 'health' to be? Many such texts on health promotion identify the wide range of concepts involved, yet most health promotion activity funded by government remains focused on a very narrow range of influences. For example, Linda Ewles and Ina Simnett's *Promoting Health*, first published in the mid-1980s and reprinted several times, has become a standard text for scores of health promotion courses, modules and training events across the UK. In very basic terms, Ewles and Simnett describe mental, emotional, social, spiritual and societal health as being at least equal concerns as physical health. These definitions have (rightly) become part of the fundamental thinking of thousands of practitioners in Britain. Yet how often does mainstream funding for health promotion activity embrace people's emotional health directly, or consider developing social networks as a *primary* aim? How much money is spent on helping people to develop their spirituality, compared to attempting to prevent coronary heart disease or HIV infection?

It is unsurprising, then, that the discrepancy between the fundamental tenets of health promotion theory and actual health promotion provision is beginning to attract criticism which, in our view, goes to the heart of health promotion theorising and model-making.

Smoking behaviour as a test of theory and models

On the popular front, the public (and corporate) response to attempts to reduce smoking is interesting to observe. The 1980s saw the rise of an organisation describing itself as the 'Freedom Organisation for the Right to Enjoy Smoking Tobacco', or FOREST. While relying on substantial funding from tobacco companies, FOREST together with several other similar groups, as well as a handful of 'celebrity' individuals, claimed to protect the rights of smokers against the activities of health promoters, frequently describing them in perjorative terms ranging from 'the health police' through to 'health fascists'. Despite the undoubted vested interests of the industry, FOREST's activities challenge what they see as the ever more strident hectoring of smokers as individuals who not only are feckless about their own health and ignorant of the risks they run, but also as a group who pollute non-smokers' bodies in a way that borders on the criminal.

We would argue that whilst FOREST's motivations may be questionable, their message should be listened to by health promoters: trying to persuade around a third of the population that what they do on a daily basis, an activity which (to themselves) is generally pleasurable, and an integral part of their lives – and to which true (deep) meaning is often attached – is in some way deviant, irresponsible and potentially the subject of litigation may not be the best method of gaining support, changing attitudes or modifying behaviour.

A more realistic model, we suggest, emerges from viewing all human behaviour as having *meaning* as well as utility. By way of illustration, cigarette smoking and recent trends in intervention provide a useful example. Smokers may well continue smoking, and find it difficult to quit, at least in part because they are dependent on nicotine. Indeed, there is now good evidence that nicotine replacement therapies can assist some smokers in quitting, at least in the short term. Yet it must also be recognised that the vast majority of people who have stopped smoking (and who have remained abstinent) in the last few decades have done so without the use of pharmaceutical help, counselling, group therapy or the benefit of so-called 'specialist' smoking cessation advisers. While such aids can increase the likelihood of an attempt to quit being successful, it remains true that the very best interventions, provided by well-trained staff, still have high failure rates and even higher relapse rates. A clue to why smoking remains a very difficult activity for some people to give up (while paradoxically most successful quitters do so alone and unaided) is provided by a brief examination of previous attempts to classify smokers into 'types'.

Early efforts to explain motivations for smoking led to the construction of a number of 'smoker typologies' in which people's reasons for smoking were categorised. This work has been used to form the basis for past intervention materials (Cancer Research Campaign/TACADE, 1988), and perhaps more importantly because these studies were precursors to later work on gender differences in smoking motivation. Several typologies have been proposed, with some models being later combined into more complex higher-order structures. However, the following four principal categories may be identified:

a) **Those based on subjective/cognitive responses**
   In this category, smokers' reasons for smoking are seen as falling into one or more groups, which reflect differing levels of 'need', ranging from stress reduction to the enhancement of pre-existing relaxation: for example, Tomkins (1966), McKennell (1970) and Coan (1973).

b) **Those based on different experienced effects**
   In this category, smokers are seen to use cigarettes in order to induce directly certain psychological effects, such as stimulation or relaxation: for example, Ikard, Green and Horn (1969), Russell, Peto and Patel (1974) and Myrsten et al. (1975).

c) **Those linking craving to empirical situations**
   In this category, smokers are viewed as smoking in response to the desire for cigarettes triggered by a specific situation, such as after meals or during breaks from work: for example, McKennell and Thomas (1967), Frith (1971), Best (1975) and O'Connor (1985).

d) **Those linking personality with empirical situations**
   Here, traditional personality variables such as extraversion or neuroticism are combined with given situations to define categories of smoking behaviour: for example, Schalling (1977) and Knott (1979).

In approaches which combine these categories, Tomkins (1968) and Ikard, Green and Horn (1969) found significantly different scores for negative affect control in female subjects compared to male subjects, a finding which stimulated further research into gender differences in smoking. Batten (1985) applied Russell et al.'s (1974) typology test to a sample of smokers taken from cessation groups and showed that women appeared to smoke more for sedative effects than did men; however, she acknowledges that the remaining analyses of her results were based on a very low response rate and may be less reliable.

Despite these early findings, most attempts to define 'types of smoker' have been largely unsuccessful in explaining variance in smoking behaviour, preventing smoking uptake or helping people quit. The main problem, we would argue, is that irrespective of how such a categorisation is framed, smokers are *people* who may smoke for different reasons at different times during the course of their smoking careers (or even at different times of day), and may thus move in and out of any of these categories from one moment to the next; this is particularly true if smoking is continued over a period of many years, during which the smoker's life circumstances may change quite fundamentally. Thus, some smokers use tobacco to regulate mood, others to relieve tension, and still others as an integral part of any enjoyable occasion.

The essential point is that smoking, a subject arguably at the top of the list of 'behaviours to be changed' in most British health promotion programmes, is not a discrete, distinct activity isolated from everyday life, the 'prevalence' (as epidemiologists would put it) of which needs to be 'reduced'. The grounding of health promotion in epidemiological values and explanations separates the human from the 'scientific' in such a way that partly explains the limited success of typical health promotion interventions and at the same time raises ethical and philosophical concerns.

Risk rules!

Førde (1998) has expressed these concerns articulately and comprehensively. He notes that preventive medicine and health promotion both have their roots in epidemiology, and through epidemiology connect to health politics in most industrialised nations. Thus Førde argues that (via health promotion activities) epidemiologists have profoundly affected our way of eating, drinking, our physical activity, our relationship with sunshine, our working environments and our sexual behaviour. However, unlike other powerful influences such as nuclear science or biotechnology, this influence has never been balanced by ethical considerations of how the epidemiologically-based 'output of everyday risks to a population [might affect] an increasing proportion of the worried well' (p. 1155).

This output has been examined carefully by Skolbekken (1995), who used Medline databases to search for journal articles with the term *risk(s)* in either the title or abstract, for the 25-year period from 1967 to 1991. He describes such papers as 'risk-articles'. In addition, separate searches were made of seven of the most widely read and prestigious medical journals from the USA, Britain and Scandinavia, as well as a number of more specialist journals. Skolbekken found that, firstly the word 'risk' had gained frequency in medical journals over the last three decades. This trend was found across all the generalist journals. Overall, the proportion of 'risk-articles' found in 1967 was 0.1%. By 1991, this proportion had risen to 10–12% in the generalist journals. In the same period, 27% of all articles registered with Medline were 'risk-articles'. Even more striking was the escalation of this trend: more than 50% of all 'risk-articles' had been published in the last five years prior to the study. Articles that discussed 'risk' (in the context in which we employ the term here) had increased sharply in journals representing all disciplines, especially in obstetrics and gynaecology. However, by far the sharpest increase was found in epidemiological journals. For example, in the *American Journal of Epidemiology*, 1.9% of contributions in the period 1967–71 were classified as 'risk-articles'. During the period 1987–91, 54.3% of contributions to that journal were found to be 'risk-articles'. Similarly, in the *International Journal of Epidemiology*, the proportions of such articles rose from 5.5% during 1972–6 to 47.6% in 1987–91.

Skolbekken describes this startling rise as a 'risk epidemic', both in terms of prevalence and contagiousness. The causes of this epidemic, he suggests are multifactorial. Firstly, there has been a general internalisation of locus of control in Western industrialised societies, but that this has taken place predominantly within professional communities. By contrast, Davison, Davey Smith and Frankel (1991) have demonstrated that fatalistic attitudes are still prevalent in lay communities.

Secondly, our increased control over nature in general has allowed for a much more optimistic view of risk; rather than uncontrollable forces which threaten us, risks can be seen simply as challenges which may be overcome. Yet the most important contribution to the risk epidemic is the development of scientific thinking itself. Notions of disease aetiology have developed from paradigms of single to multiple causation, including uncertainty as a factor.

Førde encapsulates these issues concisely and eloquently:

> This moral crusade, evolving from epidemiological research and health promotion, represents a cultural unification, which threatens even those values which are generally held in high esteem in the western world. The lower social classes, as well as many cultural minorities within our industrialized world, are not only characterized by bad health, risk taking and over indulgence, but are correspondingly marked by values such as conviviality, sharing, tolerance and sociability. It is hard to associate these values with the public health movement. If these attitudes are devalued or lost, it will ultimately affect social conventions and human interaction. The apparently obvious choice of a society with individualized responsibility and long life expectancy is no longer evident, and cannot expect general endorsement if the public or cultural minorities get an explicit and real choice. The public health and health promotion movement indisputably has a mandate to improve health. The mandate to change culture is much more open to dispute. (p. 1158)

Skolbekken (1995) echoes this idea. He suggests that a preoccupation with risk is itself detrimental to health, as it imposes an unnecessary strain and fear on individuals who are otherwise generally healthy. Moreover, as Davison et al. (1991) have demonstrated, the net result among lay people is a fatalism which is the precise opposite of what most health promoters strive to achieve. Skolbekken cites Skrabanek and McCormick's (1990) well-known suggestion that 'since life itself is a universally fatal sexually transmitted disease', living it to the full demands a balance between reasonable and unreasonable risk.

Such considerations, in our view, point to the need for a radical over-haul of the focus of health promotion that is long overdue. Health promotion as a discipline has a long history of the absorption of models and theories derived from the social sciences. Over a quarter of a century ago, Marshall Becker proposed what was to become one of the most influential models ever to be adopted by health promoters: the Health Belief Model (Becker, 1974). It is therefore telling that Becker (1993) himself has commented on the undesirability of health promotion practice being predicated on epidemiologists' calculations of population risks and ever-more strident hectoring of the general public to engage in or desist from behaviours which may or may not have an influence over their personal risk of contracting certain (expensive) diseases. We conclude this chapter with Becker's own words:

> I am most concerned about what happens to us as individuals when 'Health' becomes the paramount value of our society. Advocates of health promotion and 'wellness' claim to be striving for 'self-actualization' and 'personal fulfillment'. But theologians and philosophers have generally agreed that to attain such fulfillment one must make a commitment to something beyond one's own self – quite the opposite direction from an emphasis on personal risk factors and lifestyle. I fear that as practiced currently, health promotion fosters a dehumanizing self-concern that substitutes personal health goals for more important, humane, societal goals. It is a new religion, one in which we worship ourselves, attribute good health to our devoutness, and view illness as just punishment for those who have not yet seen the Way. ... I do not think that lowering my cholesterol is going to 'self-actualize' me. I feel certain that when Socrates said, 'The life which is unexamined is not worth living,' he was not thinking of colorectal cancer screening. For the sake of our society and of humanity in general, we must begin to turn our concerns outward. If indeed, avoiding some health risks buys some of us a few more years of life, we should be worrying about the quality of society and environment in which those years will be spent. (1993: 5)

SEVEN   The indivisibility of the individual from society

What loneliness is more lonely than distrust?

George Eliot

Loneliness and the feeling of being unwanted is the most terrible poverty.

Mother Teresa

When we arrive it is 10.30 pm, it is dark and the estate looks threatening. Someone comes out to let us into the school gates. We are introduced to three young people, who take us to a classroom to talk. Our translator explains that we are interested in the work that they do with old people. There are around 200 volunteers aged between 14 and 23 in their group, with a core of around 20 who handle all the administration. The scale of their work is astonishing. There are 2400 people aged 65 and over in Carnide, one of the poorest areas of Lisbon. This year, the young people have taken over 600 of them on holiday, raising their own funds by all manner of events and renting (and driving) an elderly coach to do it. They provide some form of organised activity at least weekly, in addition to collecting shopping, running errands, doing house repairs, going for walks, and putting on entertainment. They produce a weekly newspaper and operate a 24-hour 'on-call' rota for emergencies. Perhaps most important of all, many of their number spend a great deal of time visiting older people, befriending them and simply providing company. They do not do this as a series of one-offs: the older people present show photographs of their 'young friends', noting that although some of the youngsters who were involved in the scheme years ago now have children of their own, they still keep in contact.

We explain that work on such a scale is very rare in the UK, and ask them why they do it. Despite being far too polite to say so, it is obvious that they think this a very peculiar question to ask. They reply simply: 'Because we like it.' On gentle probing, they say, 'We like the old people. They teach us a lot, and they say that we keep them young.'

The simplicity and directness of their response is profound and utterly disarming. They just consider their activities to be normal behaviour, and are very surprised that all young people in the UK don't do the same.

Age differences and health

The age profile of Britain is changing along with those of most western industrial countries. Table 7.1 shows the nature of this change.

As we noted in Chapter 3, the change in the age profile of populations reflects greatly decreased infant mortality rather than extended lifespans. Age profiles are also influenced by gender. In Western industrial countries the sex ratio favours women but this is not the case in South Asia, where female infant mortality exceeds that of male children (Cockerham, 2001).

The foundations of health in adult life are laid in the prenatal period, infancy and early childhood and this advantages individuals born into comfortable economic circumstances. Maternal smoking and poor diet adversely affect prenatal and infant development and may reduce cardio-vascular, respiratory, kidney and pancreatic function in adulthood. When both parents smoke respiratory development is likely to be inhibited. Poverty, that results in poor nutrition and physical development, may affect parents and children alike, resulting in problems both in attachment and intellectual development (Wilkinson & Marmot, 1998). Nonetheless, the average life expectancy in the industrial world has risen throughout the 20th century as we noted above. The ageing or 'greying' of populations in industrial nations, alongside falling birth rates, poses serious questions not only concerning health but economic development as well.

Although age affects health it is difficult to separate the effects of age from those of gender, race and social class. Nonetheless, we start with a

Table 7.1 Percentage of people over 65 years of age in Britain

Decade	Percent
1971	13.3
1981	15.1
1991	15.9
2031 (Projection)	16.0+

taxonomy of the lifespan. Laslett (1989) has divided the life course into four ages. He describes these as follows:

- First age: period of education
- Second age: the working life
- Third age: retirement characterised as post working and child-rearing
- Fourth age: end of life described in terms of decline, decrepitude and death.

Of course the content of each of these ages varies with gender, race and socio-economic status. An interesting finding deriving from research on health status in the first age is the absence of a social gradient of health among adolescents. It has been argued that the influences of school, peer group and youth culture account for the greater homogeneity during this period (West, 1997).

In the second age gender and social class are important determinants of health (cf. Arber & Cooper, 2000). Using British household survey data, Arber and Cooper report that the social gradient, reflecting both education and occupation, affects men and women but that the impact of the occupational gradient is greater for men than for women during this life phase. Women are more influenced by family structure. Both men and women benefit from marriage while being a single mother puts women at greater risk of ill health than are married women or men.

There is less research on health in the third age than demographic change and the greying of populations in Western industrial countries might suggest. Arber and Cooper (2000) report surprise at the similarity of health outcomes between men and women. The social gradient is more determining than gender at this period in the life course and the last occupation before retirement is predictive of inequalities in health for men. They speculate that divorce and the resulting deprivation of divorced women may, in future, increase the effects of gender on health in this age group.

Another way to look at the data provided by epidemiologists and actuaries is to enquire whether individuals across the lifespan have subjective expectations about the lengths of their lives which match statistics produced by professionals. Mirowsky (1999) investigated this question by asking 2037 Americans between 18 and 95 years of age to estimate how many more years they expected to live. Technically, the average number of years of life for an age group is termed life expectancy by demographers.

Perhaps the most surprising finding of Mirowsky's study (1999) was his report that younger people made estimates that were closer to current mortality tables than to the projections of demographers, which suggest that young people can expect to have a longer life expectancy than the current cohort of older adults. He proposed that the life expectancies of older adults did not match those of demographers as well as younger people's expectations because continuing survival among older adults encouraged optimism about the number of years remaining. The influence of gender, social class and race upon the relationship between subjective estimates of life expectancy and professional data will be considered when we examine the influence of gender, race and social class in the sections that follow. The apparent failure of young adults to appreciate the prospect of lengthening life expectancy could provide health promotion communicators with a positive opportunity.

Gender and health

The overall picture of the relationship of gender to health suggests that there is an inverse relationship between morbidity and mortality (Cockerham, 2001). When we examined US death rates by age and sex in Table 3.2, it was clear that women in the USA live longer than men. Specifically, actuarial tables for life expectancy at all ages, and across race, show that women have greater life expectancies than do men. In the UK on average women live more than five years longer than do men. Men are more likely to die in accidents and as the result of violence, to commit suicide or die from cardiovascular disease or AIDS than are women (Archer & Lloyd, 2002).

Data from the USA suggests that women have a higher morbidity rate than do men (Cockerham, 2001). Women suffer an 11 times greater rate of acute conditions which are unrelated to pregnancy than do men. These include both infectious and parasitic diseases and respiratory ailments. The only acute category in which there are more men than women is injuries. Women also have a higher morbidity rate from chronic diseases such as hypertension, colitis, arthritis and diabetes than do men, but men tend to suffer more from chronic diseases which result in death, such as cancer.

Nonetheless, in terms of life expectancy, Mirowsky (1999) reports, both from published studies and from his own research, that men expect to live almost as long as do women. He offers two explanations for these optimistic mortality expectations. He suggests that younger men may be aware of gender differences but believe there is greater opportunity for improvement in their prospects than there are for women who already live on into considerable old age. Another possibility is that men perceive themselves to be healthier than do women. Morbidity data, mentioned in the previous paragraph, supports such a perception. In addition, men tend to have more years of education, better occupational prospects and wealth; all factors that we have identified as improving health and increasing longevity.

However, Mirowsky (1999) reports some research (Ross & Bird, 1994) which suggests better health and higher socio-economic status is associated with a greater expected gap in the life expectancy of men and women. Interestingly, Mirowsky speculates that optimism could be an escape from retirement planning rather than a platform from which economic planning could be modified.

In considering the influence of gender on health, we also need to take account of gender influences across the lifespan. In their investigations of male/female differences in health in Britain, Arber and Cooper (2000) employed the concept of time periods – childhood, working life and later life. Childhood was deemed to end when an individual reached 16 years of age. The years of working life were identified as 20–59 while later life encompassed the years beginning at 60.

We have already commented upon the general influence of social economic status (SES) on health. The indicators most commonly used to assess SES are education, family income and occupation (Herrnstein & Murray, 1994). The important new finding reported by Arber and Cooper (2000) is that the childhood morbidity of boys, defined in terms of a limiting, long-standing illness, is predicted by family work status and housing tenure but that it is not significantly related to traditional measures of SES. After examining family structure, that is, couple and lone parent families, employment and housing, they concluded that parental employment versus unemployment was the strongest factor influencing health in childhood, and that boys and girls were similarly affected by social inequalities.

Gender is complexly related to self-assessed health during working life. Social class defined in terms of an individual's occupation and educational qualifications influences the health both of men and women, but occupation is a more powerful predictor of men's reported health than that of women. Education, on the other hand, has a similar gradient for both sexes. Arber and Cooper (2000) assert that the earlier view, that married women experience greater ill health, is no longer valid. It is single mothers living in deprived material conditions, and similarly situated divorced and separated individuals, who report poor health.

Differences in the health of men and women in later life reflect the different life time experiences of the two sexes in this cohort. The effects of poverty are highlighted in Ginn and Arber's (1999) report showing that twice as many women as men over the age of 65 are totally dependent on the state pension. Two-thirds of men of that age and older have additional sources of income. Nonetheless, when sex differences are examined in terms of income, not only do those in the highest 20% report better health than do those in lower income groups, but there are fewer gender differences.

Ethnicity and health

The most extensive studies of the influence of race on health have been undertaken in the USA (Cockerham, 2001). Americans of Asian origin enjoy better health than do African Americans. Once again there is an effect of the social gradient as the difference is greatest among those living in disadvantaged circumstances. When comparisons are drawn with white Americans, both Hispanic and native Americans are seen to experience poorer health.

Mortality statistics of black and white Americans subdivided by gender provide a shocking contrast (Cockerham, 2001). The life expectancy of white women in 1997 was 79.9 years. It is no surprise to find that white men had a life expectancy of only 74.3 years and that black women might expect to live to 74.7 years. The expectancy of black men was 67.2 years: more than 12 years less than that of white women.

Mirowsky's (1999) study of the perception of life expectancy reveals both gender and racial anomalies. In his paper he reports statistically significant differences between subjective expectancies and actuarial estimates for all four categories, white and black women, and white and black men. The size of the discrepancies varies dramatically. White women underestimate their life expectancies (mean difference $= -00.71$) but individuals in the other three categories overestimate the years remaining to them. The means differences are:

- Black women =   3.89
- White men   =   3.16
- Black men   = 10.35

These statistics are indeed puzzling. It would appear that black women and both white and black men estimate their life expectancy to be that of white women.

Social cohesion and health

One of the landmark studies illustrating the significance of social cohesion in health is provided by Berkman and Syme (1979). In 1965, in Alameda County, California, they set out to determine whether there could be any relationship between social ties, isolation, loneliness, interpersonal relationships and group membership with mortality rates. A sample of 6928 adults was asked about their marital status, their contact with relatives and friends, membership of church or other religious groups, and membership of secular community groups or societies. Using self-assessment questionnaires, Berkman and Syme achieved an impressive 86% completion rate.

Table 7.2   Marital status and mortality % died, 1965–1974

	Men			
	30–49 years	50–59 years	60–69 years	p
Married	3.0	12.1	26.9	<0.001
Non-married	8.6	25.2	33.7	
	Women			
	30–49 years	50–59 years	60–69 years	p
Married	3.0	7.1	14.4	ns
Non-married	3.8	9.6	20.7	

While non-responders tended to be white, male and single or widowed, they did not differ substantially in demographic terms from the overall sample. The authors developed what they describe as a 'Contact Index' based on how many close friends an individual had, how many relatives they had that they felt close to, and how often they saw these individuals in the course of one month.

Nine years later, Berkman and Syme were able to locate 96% of their original sample; again (the remaining 4% did not differ significantly from those located). Mortality rates for the whole sample based on marital status are given in Table 7.2.

The differences in mortality rates for married and non-married men are, in our view, startling. In the youngest age group, non-married men were nearly three times more likely to die than were their married contemporaries; at age 50–59 years, non-married men were more than twice as likely to have died during the study period than were married men, and even in the oldest category (where overall mortality rates are highest) death rates in non-married men remained significantly higher. While these differences are not statistically significant in women, the trends are the same as those for men.

Using contact with friends and relatives as the independent variable, similar trends were observed. These are shown in Table 7.3.

These data are even more illustrative: in every age/sex category, there appears to be a negative correlation between the *extent* of social contact an individual experiences and the risk of death during the nine-year period of the study. Consistent with the studies of effects of religiosity on health described in Chapter 4, Berkman and Syme noted the apparent protective effect of church (or other religious group) membership as shown in Table 7.4.

While the differences in mortality rates found here are smaller than those for marital status or for social contacts, they remain statistically significant and are in the same direction as before.

Table 7.3   Contact with friends and relatives and mortality % died, 1965–1974

	Men			
Contact with friends and relatives	30–49 years	50–59 years	60–69 years	*p*
High	2.9	11.0	22.2	
Medium	3.4	14.2	24.9	<0.001
Low	5.1	14.5	40.7	
	Women			
Contact with friends and relatives	30–49 years	50–59 years	60–69 years	*p*
High	1.9	6.6	11.4	
Medium	2.9	7.6	17.0	<0.001
Low	5.4	12.3	31.0	

Table 7.4   Church membership and mortality % died, 1965–1974

	Men			
	30–49 years	50–59 years	60–69 years	*p*
Member	2.8	11.3	21.6	<0.05
Non-member	4.1	14.7	30.3	
	Women			
	30–49 years	50–59 years	60–69 years	*p*
Member	1.4	6.9	15.8	<0.05
Non-member	3.9	8.4	18.3	

From their complex data, Berkman and Syme developed what they describe as a Social Network Index (SNI). This composite measure includes the number of social ties that a person has with the relative importance of such ties. From this, individuals may be allocated within a four-category typology in which group 4 have the most social ties, and group 1 the least. For each of these categories, a relative risk ratio for mortality may then be calculated. When comparing people with the least social ties with others with the most social ties, the increased risk of mortality is striking, as shown in Table 7.5.

Given that typical estimates of relative risk for mortality due to cigarette smoking are typically around 1.8, these figures are quite remarkable.

Table 7.5   Social Network Index and relative risk ratios for mortality*

Age	Men	Women
30–49	2.5	4.6
50–59	3.2	2.1
60–69	1.8	3.0

*Figures show relative risk ratios for mortality between subjects in highest SNI category and subjects in lowest SNI category

Clearly, questions arise from these data. Perhaps most obviously, do isolated people smoke more, drink more alcohol, have a poorer diet, take less exercise, or engage in more risky behaviours generally? In order to address this question, Berman and Syme combined measures of smoking, alcohol consumption, eating habits, sleeping habits, physical activity and body weight and applied the results to their data. While they found, predictably, that their combined measure was associated with both mortality and their Social Network Index, *differences in mortality rates were only slightly diminished when controlling for all these known risk factors combined.*

A central theme of this book is that health promotion should be focused more on improving people's quality of life, rather than simply attempting to reduce the rates of death from certain diseases. Yet even using this latter strategy as a rationale for health promotion activity, the indication for developing programmes which improve people's social lives and which strengthen community ties is clear. Even if the risks of being socially isolated are only *half* those suggested by Berkman and Syme's data, then reductions in mortality comparable to those claimed for reducing smoking, improving diet and reducing physical inactivity may be expected from interventions which simply provide social contact. The effects of such interventions should, according to this study at least, be most prominent among women. Nevertheless, it seems unlikely that the setting up of projects *which have such outcomes as a primary aim* will be viewed as a government priority when funding reviews hold that 'individuals are ultimately responsible for their own and their children's health'.

Almost 10 years after the Berkman and Syme study, House, Landis and Umberson (1988) carried out a review of prospective studies in which they assessed the link between social support and mortality across a range of published findings. Although the earlier Berkman and Syme (1979) investigation had used only self-report data to measure individuals' health at the beginning of their research, other studies which were included in House et al.'s survey used baseline medical data. They concluded that, beyond a doubt, the lack of social relationships is a risk factor for mortality and is as strong as smoking. In particular they noted that being married is beneficial to health and that being widowed is detrimental to health. Men suffered more when widowed than did women.

Psychophysiological explanations

These clear findings raise important questions about the processes which link low social support and mortality and, indeed, strong social networks with longevity. How may social support or contact with friends and relatives protect against disease? Conversely, why should people who are socially isolated be at greater risk of morbidity and mortality?

House, Landis and Umberson state that 'social relationships appear to have generally beneficial effects on health, not solely or even primarily attributable to their buffering effects' (1988: 543). Thus an explanation which includes biological, psychological and social factors is required and it needs to go beyond the notion that social support simply ameliorates existing health problems.

House, Landis and Umberson (1988) suggest a psychophysiological theory which they assert is consistent with early developmental data, and even evolutionary data, about the survival value of social relationships. The theory which they draw upon was put forward by Bovard and proposes that:

> social relationships and contacts, mediated through the amygdala, activate the anterior hypothalamic zone (stimulating release of human growth hormone) and inhibit the posterior hypothalamic zone (and hence secretion of andrenocorticotropic hormone, cortisol, catecholamines, and associated sympathetic autonomic activity). (p. 542)

In less technical language, positive social relationships stimulate the production of a health-promoting hormone and block the production of hormones usually related to stress. More importantly for our purposes, House, Landis and Umberson identify the need to investigate the factors which determine levels of exposure to social contacts.

The nature of interventions which might effectively lower the prevalence of relative social isolation is perhaps a more difficult problem to solve. Trend analysis predicts that in the 21st century, changes in marriage and child-bearing will leave more old people without spouses or children, the major sources of social relationships. We appear to have come full circle and returned to the story of 'George' in Chapter 4.

Social isolation and sense of coherence

As we discussed briefly in Chapter 4, it is also possible that social networking and social support contribute to an individual's Sense of Coherence (SOC). Antonovsky (1979) first proposed that an individual's SOC is determined by their assessment of life as comprehensible, manageable and meaningful. More recently, he suggested that SOC is:

> a global orientation to the world, perceiving it, to a greater or lesser extent, as comprehensible, manageable and meaningful. ... It is, I submit, a central dispositional orientation in the lives of all human beings. (Antonovsky, 1987: 19)

He proposes that:

1. people throughout the life career confront a variety of tasks shaped by biological, historical and psychosocial forces;
2. the more successful they are in resolving these tasks, the more likely they are to maintain or improve their places on the health ease/dis-ease continuum; and
3. SOC is a major determinant of such success.

Clearly, high levels of perceived social support and strong social networks are likely to contribute positively to how comprehensible, manageable and meaningful an individual sees their world as being. Antonovsky (1993) views this as a dynamic process:

> The strength of [an individual's] SOC begins to be shaped well before kindergarten. By the time we have become stably functioning adults ... this dispositional orientation has largely been set. One's interpersonal and work experiences, *shaped in a framework of one's social class, gender and ethnic group membership at a given time in history,* have done their work. ... Thus, by the time one is elderly, I doubt that much change is to be anticipated. Those of us with a strong SOC will continue ... those of us who are less fortunate will increasingly see the world as incomprehensible, unmanageable and meaningless. (1993: 3)

Thus, Antonovsky hypothesised that a person who sees his/her life as meaningful and comprehensible is able to deal more successfully with health-threatening stressful situations and events. Moreover, SOC is not simply a personal construct: it is a social concept, which develops more positively among people growing up in a stable environment with clearly defined norms and values.

Lundberg and Nyström Peck (1994) explored the relationship of SOC to demographic variables and to ill health in the Swedish population. Data were collected in 1981 and again in 1991. Psychosocial variables measured in 1981 were then used to predict the likelihood of an individual having a low SOC 10 years later. Younger people were less likely than were older people to develop a low SOC; in addition, the authors demonstrated a negative relationship between socio-economic status and the odds ratio of developing low SOC in the future. More important in the current context is their finding that people who had a low SOC were 80% more likely to develop circulatory problems than were people with a high SOC. Further, people with a low SOC were 300% more likely to develop psychological problems than were their contemporaries who had a higher SOC.

Lundberg and Nyström Peck conclude that:

1. the observed relationship is likely to be causal
2. having a high SOC may be protective against circulatory and psychological problems, and
3. SOC is both internally and externally determined.

This last point is important because if SOC is partly determined by external circumstances, then it may be susceptible, in principle, to intervention.

Models of social support and disease prevention

Moving on from morbidity studies, Sheldon Cohen (1988) set out to identify the mechanism through which social support systems influence the onset of physical disease. To try and explicate these processes, Cohen examined various 'conceptions of social support', listing the processes identified as influencing health and well-being. The influence of social support is restricted to the onset and progression of physical illness.

In differentiating social support, Cohen identifies the most frequently used measures as a structural index of social ties described as social integration (SI) and functional measures. An SI index usually includes marital status, close family and friends, group activities and church/religious affiliations. Functional measures include work satisfaction and perceived availability of material and psychological support.

The most famous studies employing SI show that when traditional risk factors – high blood pressure, smoking, and cholesterol – are controlled for, a healthy person with higher SI scores is at a lower risk of dying than are individuals who are isolated. This is particularly true for men, but in women SI effects have been found to have an influence on their risk of ischemic heart disease, and on mortality among elderly (70–80-year-old) women. SI effects are stronger for Caucasian people, and are also predictive of survival among men who suffer a myocardial infarction. Marital satisfaction and satisfaction with social activities did not seem to be related to mortality, but in older adults perceived adequacy of social support was related to mortality.

Mortality statistics are silent on whether social support influences the incidence, severity, progression of, or recovery from, disease. Studies of patients with myocardial infarction suggest that social integration plays a role in progression and recovery. However, simple prevalence studies of SI and illness are open to criticism of reverse causation: that is, illness results in smaller, less accessible social networks.

Cohen's models focus on the role of social support in the onset, severity and progression of disease. He identifies three such models:

- Generic models
- Stress-centred models
- Psychosocial process models

Generic and stress-centred models appeared early on, and are relatively simple. The later psychosocial process models built on these, and specified the complexity of psychosocial details. These models are described in turn below.

Generic models

The first generic model of how social isolation may influence disease is straightforward: it views social support (or the lack of it) as influencing familiar health behaviours such as smoking, alcohol consumption, diet and exercise.

The second generic model is more complex: it suggests that support (or the lack of it) impacts on the biological responses that influence disease. Biological responses influenced by social support include neuroendocrine responses, immune responses (either directly or through neuroendocrine reactivity), and haemodynamic responses. Specifically, increased support has been held to suppress neuroendocrine and haemodynamic responses, and to increase immune competence. Conversely, diseases associated with the immune response include infectious diseases, allergies, autoimmune diseases and cancers.

These two models may be combined when the effects of behaviour are mediated by a biological response. Active forms of coping may result in increased neuroendocrine responses that may either directly or indirectly be linked to disease through the immune system. Poor diet may raise serum cholesterol levels.

Stress-centred models

Two kinds of models have been employed to explain the relationship of social support and disease outcomes. The first, known as the stress buffering model (Casel, 1976), suggests that social support is either only (or at least primarily) important for persons who are under stress. Conversely, the main effect model notes no interaction between stress and support, claiming that social support, on its own, is a positive factor regardless of stress levels. In both cases, support is linked to disease outcomes via behavioural or biological processes.

Psychosocial process models

These models rely upon the conception of specific links between support and psychosocial and biological processes as we noted above in discussing the work of House, Landis and Umberson (1988). There is sufficient empirical evidence to sustain a review of two aspects of social support. These aspects are *social integration* and the *perceived availability* of support. There is evidence for separate links of social integration (SI) and perceived availability of support in the psychosocial model. In a 30-month, prospective study of Americans of 65 years and older, Blazer (1982) found evidence that SI measures, frequency of interaction and perceived avail-ability of support all were associated with positive changes in self-care over the study period.

High levels of social support have also been linked to positive affect, and may thus protect against distress from life events associated with high stress. Two hypotheses are popularly suggested as to how social support may influence stress in individuals. First, the *direct effect hypothesis* proposes that others may intervene to reduce the *amount* of stress that a person experiences. Second, the *buffering hypothesis* suggests that social support may assist an individual in coping with the *experience* of stress. Thus, the presence of other people enables a stressed individual to draw on their experiences in order to select the most appropriate strategy for dealing with his/her own stressors.

Of course, it is possible that both these hypotheses may be true. In either case, one important outcome may be the mediation of the link between stress and consequent illness.

While many of the studies described above speculate on how social support may operate, fewer consider precisely what it might be. As a definition of social support, we favour Salovey and Rothman's (2003) suggestion that the term may be seen as 'the experience, emanating from other people, that one is valued, respected, cared about and loved' (p. 215).

It seems clear that health promotion agencies have a role to play both in the direct provision of social support to individuals, and in fostering and developing social support networks within communities. Compared to interventions aimed at reducing smoking, improving diet and encouraging exercise, such work is currently underdeveloped. We suggest that developing projects which attempt to improve people's sense of being valued, respected and cared for might well prove to be a sound investment in their future health.

EIGHT   Human perspectives in health promotion

Happiness is that state of consciousness which proceeds from the achievement of one's values.

Ayn Rand

Taking health promotion forward

In this concluding chapter, we attempt to draw together the threads which run through our preceding discussions. Here, we try to set out some kind of vision as to how health promotion might develop into a more inclusive, more holistic and, hopefully, a more effective activity than has hitherto been the case. In order to achieve this aim, we believe it is necessary for health promotion activity to be moulded on principles which more realistically reflect people's everyday lives in early 21st-century Britain. In order to do this, we propose that a shift in the way in which health promotion activity is planned, prioritised, implemented and evaluated is needed.

We begin by revisiting an important observation touched on only briefly in Chapter 3. Marmot et al.'s (1978) study of British civil servants contains data of critical importance, whose ramifications are seldom given appropriate prominence in planning health promotion strategies. It will be recalled that while Marmot's subjects displayed a gradient of morbidity with social class which mirrored trends which are now all too familiar, the effect of traditional 'health-related behaviours' such as smoking, drinking and lack of exercise only accounted for a small proportion of the variation observed. This finding is consistent with many others described earlier in this volume: Lisa Berkman's seminal work on social isolation and mortality showed an inverse relationship between meaningful social connections and death rates (Berkman & Syme, 1979). Once again, controlling for 'risk' factors such as smoking and obesity reduced the strength of the observed trend only marginally.

Health promotion activity should be guided, we suggest, not by medical practitioners who (quite reasonably) desire to reduce the prevalence of diseases. Doctors should, in our view, focus their attention on what they are expert in: the treatment of disease. In expressing this view, is not our intention to indulge in what has become popularly known (not least among health promoters) as 'doctor-bashing', but simply to point out that the undeniable rigours of the medical school curriculum have a different focus to that needed for successful health promotion planning. Similarly, developing effective health promotion strategies cannot be undertaken solely by social psychologists, although they may provide valuable contributions to understanding health-related behaviours. Above all, it is important to make it clear that we are not arguing against the desirability of programmes intended, for example, to prevent smoking uptake or to help smokers quit; neither are we suggesting that interventions aimed at improving people's diet or promoting physical activity are not of value. Clearly, it is important that the incidence of avoidable diseases be reduced, together with their concomitant pain, unhappiness and premature death rates. We do not deny that such programmes have their part to play.

Instead, we suggest that a different, *additional* approach is needed. Such an approach pays much greater respect to lay concepts of health. It may, therefore, value emotional health over the absence of physical disease; social well-being over fitness; spirituality over smoking cessation. It is these values to which we attach the collective term 'human perspectives'. By human perspectives in health promotion, we mean taking as a starting point the desire to *improve the quality of people's lives without necessarily adopting disease prevention as a **primary** aim.*

Providing initiatives based on these principles requires courage on the part of both planners and providers, and at every stage of the process. At the planning stage, it will be necessary to take heed of the rapidly growing body of evidence which could only be touched upon in the earlier chapters of this book. There is a pressing need for systematic reviews of many of the topics for which we have only provided an illustration of some possibilities. While the contribution of academics in this matter will be valuable, it is also necessary to consult 'ordinary' people about what *they* think would improve the quality of their lives, and, even more importantly, to act upon their responses, even if these do not conform to government-determined 'priorities'. It is entirely possible that such ordinary people based programmes are not amenable to the setting of 'targets' in the manner so popular with current politicians. It is a difficult and complex, but vital task to develop ways in which ordinary people may feel more valued as individuals and encouraged to express themselves more creatively. It will be an equally difficult and complex task to enable alienated people to find some sense of purpose and meaning, and to foster more integrated, functioning communities, particularly in our isolating society. The rebuilding of a more *healthy* society, as opposed to one with a lower prevalence of certain diseases, may be a gradual and protracted task.

Throughout this book, we have asserted that it is people's social environment, their emotional well-being, social interaction and 'wholeness' that determine their health status and that these should be the domains in which health promotion, as opposed to preventive medicine, should operate.

Tarlov's (1996) important work summarises evidence supporting the view that social factors are the paramount determinants of health; most importantly, he provides an explanatory framework as to why social hierarchies cause differential vulnerability to disease. In order to do this, Tarlov argues, it is necessary to return yet again to the fundamental issue with which we began this book: that is, *what is this quality called health that we are trying to promote?*

Tarlov notes that three conceptual components emerge from 50 years of debating this question. Firstly, that health is a *capacity to perform* and is thus a continuous variable, a relative state. Secondly, this capacity to perform is used to achieve *individual fulfilment*, the nature of which is determined by one's values, needs, aspirations and potential. Thirdly, good health provides the potential to effectively *negotiate the demands of the social environment* in which individuals live and within which capacity operates and fulfilment may be achieved. *Health may thus be seen as the capacity for individual fulfilment within a social context.*

Taken together, Tarlov defines health as:

> The capacity, relative to potential and aspirations, for living fully in the social environment. … The definition emphasises 'living fully'. Death and morbidity rates, the principal measures of health worldwide, are only indirect and perhaps not highly sensitive indicators of a population's health. The 3.7 years longer life expectancy of the Japanese, and the 2.1 years of the Swedish … may underestimate the true health differences if capacity for living fully in the social environment were measured. (p. 72)

Thus, Tarlov sees any given population's health at any time in history as being the net result of the interaction of people with their social and physical environment. Because the social and physical environment changes with time, so do the determinants of the health of the contemporary population. Our latter-day decline in mortality due to infectious diseases has been accompanied by a reciprocal rise in mortality from chronic diseases but also with an extraordinary increase in life expectancy. At the same time, inequalities in health status have become both more pronounced and more finely stratified. In the UK, this increasingly detailed gradient of health status with wealth mirrors the increasingly complex social stratification started by the industrial revolution, and which still exists today. Most importantly from the perspective of this book is the consistent observation that *only a small proportion* of this observed gradient can be explained by differences in health-related behaviours.

Tarlov suggests that an important contributor to this unexplained variance in health status lies in an individual's identity. Certainly, social identity can be a powerful contributor to variation in health-related behaviours, especially among adolescents (Lloyd, Lucas & Fernbach, 1997; Lucas & Lloyd, 1999; Lloyd & Lucas, 1998). Tarlov goes further, and suggests that it is the interaction of identity with environment that produces the most substantial inequalities in health. He argues that identity begins to form early in life, perhaps at around 2 to 3 years of age, and its formation may be completed in an individual's late teens. From then on, the *expectations* which flow from an individual's identity interact most powerfully with his or her environment. Specifically, observations of inequity, limitations in job opportunities, housing, income, employment stability and social segregation clash with expectations derived from identity.

The result, Tarlov argues, is a 'chronic, persistent [and] inescapable dissonance between what a person would like to do or become, and what seems accomplishable'. This dissonance in turn triggers a series of biological responses which are the antecedents of chronic disease development. The precise nature of the disease so produced depends upon genetic and other factors, so that one individual may develop atherosclerosis, while another may develop diabetes, and so on. Further, as people in any particular socio-economic group may (on average) experience broadly similar degrees of dissonance, then their potential health status might be expected to be similarly affected.

At the time of writing, empirical support for Tarlov's model is limited, but much work is in progress (e.g., Goodman et al., 2000; Goodman, 2002). Nevertheless, it does provide useful pointers for health promotion interventions of the kind we have encouraged in this volume.

In a consistent manner, many of the studies of religiosity and health discussed in Chapter 4 demonstrate the substantial contribution made by factors *other* than traditional health-related behaviours to variations in health status and mortality rates. It is remarkable enough that Levin and Schiller's (1987) review demonstrated that when comparing religious groups, there appears to be a relatively lower risk of illness in more behaviourally strict religions or denominations. Moreover, there is a clear trend towards better health, lower morbidity and lower mortality rates among people with higher levels of religiosity. But it is more remarkable still that this relationship is weakened only slightly when differences in the prevalence of 'risky' behaviours among such people are taken into account.

At the same time, it is instructive to consider mortality rates and life expectancy in the context of developed nations such as the UK. A baby boy born today in the UK can expect to live, on average, for over 81 years. His sister can expect to outlive him and reach an age of over 84 years (ONS, 2004). Of course, these figures are crude means which hide a range of lifespans with some less fortunate citizens dying far earlier, and some (though not necessarily more fortunate) people living far longer. In 1932, there were 320 known centenarians in the UK. In 2003, there were over 8000. Yet while some contemporary differences in longevity are attributable to individual behaviours, much of this difference cannot be so explained and is influenced (or even determined) by factors that are completely beyond individual control or choice. Taken together, these observations and those of many similar studies demonstrate the magnitude of the effects of psychosocial factors in the development of physical disease, and conversely of psychological well-being in promoting health.

The effects of dislocation, unemployment, bereavement and stress generally have long been accepted as pathogenic. We believe that the salutogenic effects of a sense of coherence, social cohesion, inclusion, and feelings of purpose and meaning have been given far too little consideration, particularly by those planning, commissioning and delivering public health policies. The implementation of any initiative planned on such principles does not necessarily require 'expert' supervision, at least not in the conventional sense of the word. The expertise required for the successful working of such programmes lies not in academic or professional qualifications, but in a more intimate, empathetic and emotionally intelligent involvement of the participants involved. Specifically, it necessitates a certain relinquishing of professional power. Hawe and Shiell (2000) make this point clearly:

> Not only is power and powerlessness implicated as a variable in the production of health inequalities ... but practitioners who seek to promote health have been conscious of the way they work, lest they reinforce status hierarchies. ... even common methods of needs assessment in a community can act simply to reinforce the status quo. (p. 879)

If the determinants of health vary with changing social circumstances, then it follows that strategies to improve health will also change over time. We suggest, therefore, that not only the planning and prioritisation of health promotion strategies needs to be reviewed. The manner in which health promotion activity is delivered would, in our view, benefit from consideration of Tarlov's work, and particularly that of Lisa Berkman, described in Chapter 7.

If the planning and implementation of health promotion activity is to change, then different measures need to be developed to evaluate its effectiveness. Although many attempts have been made to evaluate existing health promotion programmes, the benefits of evaluation in health promotion to date may best be described as mixed. On the one hand, evaluation is an important activity: it is obviously helpful to audit health promotion programmes in terms of effectiveness in order to inform future projects. On the other hand, there has been enormous pressure on health promoters in recent years to address the question 'Does it actually work?' We believe that this pressure has been unhelpful for two reasons.

First, few areas of health or social intervention have been subject to so much scrutiny, by so many masters, in proportion to their allotted funding. Despite considerable improvements in the last few years, health promotion departments still receive a comparatively small proportion of NHS funding. Nevertheless, the level of supervision they have attracted in terms of committees, steering groups, advisory panels and senior management (often by public health doctors) is, in our experience, quite disproportionate to their size, budget and staffing levels. This has had a number of effects on those delivering health promotion programmes. In general, there has been an emphasis on outcomes which are quantifiable, repeatable and, perhaps above all, easy to measure. Second, the resultant 'beancounting' approach to evaluation provides little insight as to *why* a particular intervention succeeds or fails. Moreover, despite the fact that much health promotion activity is currently aimed at changing individual behaviour, few projects have the funding, expertise or even (given the serial changes in NHS organisational structures in the last two decades) adequate continuity of management to assess changes in anything other than the short term.

If we are interested in improving people's quality of life, then we need to place much greater emphasis on more appropriate ways of measuring our success. By 'appropriate', we mean methods which measure directly the kinds of outcomes we are trying to achieve. If, for example, we wish to improve social cohesion and inclusion, then we need to measure how much people feel a part of their community, rather than, say, counting how many people attend a particular organised group. As Hawe and Shiell (2000) point out, fostering a sense of community has been a primary goal of community psychology since the early 1970s (Sarason, 1974). For this reason, the measurement of 'sense of community' as a construct is well established (Davidson & Cotter, 1986). Nevertheless, and despite the seeming ubiquity of rhetoric concerning social capital, 'sense of community' is a variable found rarely among the many maps of health and disease which make up the statutory reports produced annually by every Director of Public Health in the UK. Similarly, if we wish to measure improvements in local people's mental well-being – as opposed to 'reducing the incidence of depression in the community' – then we need to explore sensitively how they feel about themselves and their lives, rather than counting prescriptions for Prozac.

Inevitably, measuring these kinds of outcomes requires different kinds of expertise in evaluation than those available to most current health promotion programmes. Currently, few public health departments are fortunate enough to have many individuals skilled in qualitative research. Roberts, Towell and Golding (2001: 255) note the growing respect afforded to qualitative methods which offer 'a unique route for exploring questions of meaning in both quality-of-life research and that concerning the nature and role of social relationships'. They go on to suggest that such techniques may be of particular assistance in understanding in what ways social inequalities result in inequalities in health status, and point to Tarlov's work described above. Moreover, from the point of view of health promotion research, the authors suggest two ways in which qualitative methodologies are particularly valuable. Firstly, such methods 'put flesh on the bones' of existing models, so that they give concrete *meaning* to abstract statistical models. This contribution is, in our view, an essential adjunct to help address the limitations of social-psychological models of health promotion discussed in Chapter 5. Secondly, qualitative methods provide an evidence-based platform from which to generate more rigorously testable hypotheses about the determinants of health and health-related behaviours. Roberts et al. (2001) summarise this approach eloquently:

> [Qualitative methodology] might not always provide a *de rigueur* objective account of verifiable processes in the material world, but on occasion it is the only and therefore the best available form of data for empirical investigations of meaning and self-determination in human affairs. Where this is the case ... it should be considered that human testimony possesses intrinsic validity. (p. 255)

The Emperor's New Clothes?

If health promotion is to be as 'evidence based' as many of its proponents would wish, then we must first face some fairly unpalatable facts. First, much ill health is not preventable solely by the familiar targets of health promotion campaigns. Second, such campaigns have, if we are brutally honest, been pretty unsuccessful in achieving their aims. Overall rates of smoking, for example, have decreased only slightly in the last decade, and among some groups (ironically those most exposed to health promotion interventions, such as children) rates have actually increased alarmingly. Overall the use of illegal drugs continues to rise, alcohol dependence is increasingly common among the young, while obesity is said to be reaching 'epidemic' levels. Put bluntly, the 'evidence' is that much health promotion, as practised currently, simply doesn't work.

So where do we go from here? We have suggested a fundamental shift of the criteria upon which health promotion activities in the UK are decided. We suggest that determining priorities for health promotion should pass from the hands of public health doctors, epidemiologists and government policy-makers to the hands of those to whom health promotion campaigns are currently directed: ordinary people. Many textbook authors, academics, researchers and health promotion workers have been driven by notions of 'empowerment'. Yet this term has become so over-used (and often poorly defined by health promoters) that Raeburn and Rootman (1998) have noted in exasperation:

> Empowerment is not a word we like all that well. It is unquestionably a (if not *the*) current 'buzz word' in health promotion and community development ... but like all over-used words, one can get tired of hearing it or it tends to be misused or misunderstood. (p. 64)

These authors go on to note that there is a distinct scarcity of literature which describes what the experience is actually like from the perspective of the individual who is 'empowered', despite the volume of writing (and, we would add, the hundreds of professional conferences, seminars, committees, 'partnerships' and 'action groups') which concern themselves with empowerment. Even in those studies which have focused on such experiences, the primary factor of study seems to have been confined to an increase in the sense of personal control (Lord & Farlow, 1990). This is hardly surprising given that participants were selected on the basis of having increased control over their lives, and that they were subsequently interviewed about precisely this issue.

Yet Lord and Farlow's findings go to the heart of health promotion principles. Firstly, their respondents saw having the power to define *their own* needs as being key to the process of their own empowerment. Secondly, the assumption that individuals might actually understand their own needs better than do 'experts' driven by professional, epidemiological and political imperatives is one which is not generally popular with those professionals and politicians who formulate health promotion policy, and who decide on health promotion priorities. It appears that health promoters wish to 'empower' ordinary people, but only provided that such empowerment results in them changing to behaviours which experts consider appropriate. Rappaport (1981) described this subterfuge forcefully:

> Prevention programmes aimed at so-called high-risk populations, especially programmes under the auspices of established social institutions, can easily become a new arena for colonisation, where people are forced to consume our goods and services, thereby providing us [professionals] with jobs and money. (pp. 12–13)

Yet almost 25 years on, such programmes continue to be promulgated, despite the absence of evidence for their effectiveness. On the very day that this page was written (February 2004), the Royal Colleges of Physicians, Paediatrics and Child Health, together with the Faculty of Public Health Medicine, vociferously urged the British government to launch a campaign to reduce levels of obesity in the UK. Under the banner heading 'Reducing and Preventing Obesity: Everything must Change', the RCP introduced their report *Storing up Problems: The Medical Case for a Slimmer Nation* (RCP, 2004). At pains not to exclude anyone, the report proclaims that 'action needs to be taken at every possible level – national, local, community and as individuals'. It recommends that a 'cross-governmental task force should be established at Cabinet level' in order to 'develop national strategies for tackling the threat from overweight and obesity', and demands 'a sustained public education campaign to improve people's understanding of the benefits of healthy eating and active living'. In a curiously oxymoronic manner, it proposes that 'Population-wide initiatives should be implemented at local level' to tackle obesity. Apart from the somewhat chilling exhortation ('Everything must Change'), we believe such proposals are as unfocused as they are patronising and lacking a firm evidence base. It seems very likely to us that given the pervasiveness of mass advertising, television 'lifestyle' programmes, certain food manufacturers and the sports and fitness industries, most adults in the UK probably have some notion of 'the benefits of healthy eating and active living' and probably do not need to be told about them yet again.

By contrast, we believe that what may enable people to make changes to their eating habits may have little, if anything, to do with 'understanding the benefits' to be had from whatever 'active living' may mean. Fifteen years ago, Lord and Farlow noted that people's empowerment to make change depended most crucially on *being involved in community life* in the manner they considered appropriate for them:

> What we found ... was that regardless of the nature of the participation – whether it was based on common recreational or cultural interests, political concerns, or the desire for mutual support – simply being accepted as a member of the group was an important factor for many people. (p. 7)

As Raeburn and Rootman (1998) observe, among all the social factors impacting on empowerment, *participation in community activity* is the single most important contribution to the development of a sense of empowerment.

Seen in this light, the work of the Peckham Health Centre, so many years ago, suddenly does not seem so dated. People's medical needs were attended to, health education [sic] was provided and exercise encouraged, but crucially these activities took place in the context of providing recreation, social interaction and a focus point for the local community.

We have maintained that traditional health promotion initiatives have relied too heavily on the notion of beliefs and attitudes determining behaviour. One reason for the failure of such approaches to explain why people do or do not do certain things (or 'perform behaviours', to use the language of health promoters) is that attitudes and beliefs by themselves do not account for the influence of emotions in decision-making processes. Hence it may be more illuminating to consider *values,* rather than just knowledge and attitudes. We see values not simply as beliefs, but as *culturally-mediated and emotionally-charged* beliefs which may be much more influential on health-related behaviours than simple cognitions.

If we ask people about their values, and what they believe would improve the quality of their lives most, how might they answer? These are not questions that have been extensively or systematically studied by academics, at least not in the UK. Such studies that are available are fairly superficial in nature and often demonstrate considerable bias because they are conducted by political, corporate or single-interest groups. Nevertheless, we are reasonably confident that safety, reducing crime, improving community relations, and having adequate social, recreational and cultural facilities are likely to feature more prominently than 'tackling obesity levels', 'improving cardiovascular fitness' or banning cigarette smoking.

Based on a number of such studies in Canada, Raeburn and Rootman (1998) report that, despite there being no single articulated set of values among those they describe as 'ordinary people', a broad consensus of opinion does seem to exist among their respondents. They describe their findings as:

> the desire to do well by one's children, the wish to contribute meaningfully to society, the desire to have opportunities to get together with others at the community level, the wish to help those who are incapacitated or otherwise temporarily or permanently at a disadvantage, the wish for respect and dignity to be shown towards oneself and also to show that to others, the wish to be loved or at least respected by others, the desire for a sense of community, the wish for a pleasant community environment with good facilities, the desire to acquire new knowledge and skills regardless of age, and the desire for a 'fair deal' for everyone. (p. 217)

The authors remark that these values emerge with extraordinary consistency in every study they have performed, and that these shared values seem to span all classes, all cultures and all age groups. If we are to produce a healthier society, we believe this would be a good place to start.

References

Abraham, C. & Sheeran, P. (2003a). Implications of goal theories for the theories of reasoned action and planned behaviour. *Current Psychology, 22*, 264–280.

Abraham, C. & Sheeran, P. (2003b). Acting on intentions: The role of anticipated regret. *British Journal of Social Psychology, 42*, 495–511.

Abraham, C., Sheeran, P., Norman, P., Conner, M., de Vries, N. & Otten, W. (1999). When good intentions are not enough: Modelling postdecisional cognitive correlates of condom use. *Journal of Applied Social Psychology, 29*, 2591–2612.

Aggleton, P. (1994). *Health*. London and New York: Routledge.

Aggleton, P. & Homans, H. (1987). *Educating about AIDS*. London: National Health Service.

Aho, W.R. (1979). Participation of senior citizens in the swine flu inoculation program: An analysis of health belief model variables in preventive health behavior. *Journal of Gerontology, 34*, 201–208.

Ainsworth, S. (1999). A plague on public health. *Health Service Journal*, 7 January.

Ajzen, I. (1998). Models of human social behaviour and their application to health psychology. *Psychology and Health, 13*, 735–739.

Ajzen, I. & Fishbein, M. (Eds.) (1980). *Understanding attitudes and predicting social behavior*. Englewood Cliffs, NJ: Prentice-Hall.

Ajzen, I. & Madden, T.J. (1986). Prediction of goal-directed behaviour: Attitudes, intentions and perceived behavioral control. *Journal of Experimental Social Psychology, 22*, 453–474.

Allen, D.T. (1997). Effects of dogs on human health. *Journal of the American Veterinary Medicine Association, 210*, 1136–1139.

Anderson, W., Reid, C. & Jennings, G. (1992). Pet ownership and risk factors for cardio-vascular disease. *Medical Journal of Australia, 157*, 298–301.

Antonovsky, A. (1979). *Health, stress and coping: New perspectives on mental and physical well-being*. San Francisco: Jossey-Bass.

Antonovsky, A. (1987). *Unravelling the mystery of health*. San Francisco: Jossey-Bass.

Antonovsky, A. (1993). *The salutogenic approach to ageing*. Address to University of California, Berkeley, 21st January 1993. www.angelfire.com/ok/soc/a-berkeley.html

Arber, S. & Cooper, H. (1999). Gender differences in later life: the new paradox. *Social Science & Medicine, 48*, 61–76.

Arber, A. & Cooper, H. (2000). Gender and inequalities in health across the lifecourse. In E. Annandale & K. Hunt (Eds.), *Gender inequalities in health* (pp. 123–149). Buckingham and Philadelphia: Open University Press.

Archer, J. & Lloyd, B. (2002). *Sex and gender* (2nd edn). Cambridge: Cambridge University Press.

Aronowitz, R.A. (1998). *Making sense of illness: Science, society and disease*. Cambridge: Cambridge University Press.

Armitage, C.J. & Conner, M. (2001). Efficacy of the theory of planned behaviour: A meta-analytic review. *British Journal of Social Psychology, 40*, 471–499.

Atkinson, P. (1995). Medical talk and medical work: The liturgy of the clinic. *American Journal of Epidemiology, 115*, 684–694.

Bäckman, G. (1990). Life control and perceived health. *Tijdschr Soc Gezondheidsz*, Suppl. 11: 123–127.

Bäckman, G. (1991). Livskontroll – en buffert mot ohälsa? (Life control – a buffer against ill health?) In B. Bergsten, A. Bjerkmans, H.-E. Hermanssohn & J. Israel (Eds.), *Etik, Solidaritet, Välfärd. Festskrift till Harald Swedner* (Ethics, Solidarity, Welfare. Festschrift for Harald Swedner) (pp. 231–237). Uddevalla: Diadalos.

Bailey, S.L., Ennett, S.T. & Ringwalt, C.L. (1993). Potential mediators, moderators, or independent effects in the relationship between parents' former and current cigarette use and their children's cigarette use. *Addictive Behaviors, 18*, 601–621.

Bandura, A. (1977). Self-efficacy: Toward a unifying theory of behaviour change. *Psychological Review, 84*, 191–215.

Batten, L. (1985). *Addiction and perceived dependence as smoking motivations: An empirical analysis*. Unpublished manuscript, University of Southampton, UK.

Bauman, K. (1987). School of Public Health, University of Carolina, USA. In D. Mcvey (Ed.), *Teenage smoking: A report on an expert seminar examining the use of mass-media strategies to reduce smoking among teenagers*. London: HEA.

Beck, U. (1992). *Risk society: Towards a new modernity*. London: Sage.

Becker, M.H. (1974). The health belief model and personal health behaviour. *Health Education Mongraphs, 2*, 324–508.

Becker, M.H. (1993). A medical sociologist looks at health promotion. *Journal of Health and Social Behaviour, 34*, 1–6.

Becker, M.H. & Rosenstock, I.M. (1984). Compliance with medical advice. In A. Steptoe & A. Mathews (Eds.), *Health care and human behaviour*. London: Academic Press.

Belsky, J. (1980). Child maltreatment: An ecological integration. *American Psychologist, 34*, 320–335.

Belsky, J. (1984). The determinants of parenting: A process model. *Child Development, 55*, 83–96.

Benjamin, J. (1998). *The shadow of the other: Intersubjectivity and gender in psychoanalysis*. New York and London: Routledge.

Bennett, L.W., Cardone, S. & Jarczyk, J. (1998). Effects of a therapeutic camping program on addiction recovery: The Algonquin Relapse Prevention Program. *Journal of Substance Abuse Treatment, 15*, 469–474.

Bentler, P.M. & Speckart, G. (1979). Models of attitude-behaviour relations. *Psychological Review, 86*, 452–464.

Berger, P.L. & Luckman, T. (1967). *The social construction of reality*. London: Allen Lane.

Berkman, L.F. & Syme, S.L. (1979). Social networks, host resistance and mortality: A nine year follow-up study of Alameda County residents. *American Journal of Epidemiology, 109*, 186–204.

Berman, D.S. & Anton, M.T. (1988). A wilderness therapy program as an alternative to adolescent psychiatric hospitalisation. *Residential Treatment Children and Youth, 5*, 41–53.

Best, J.A. (1975). Tailoring smoking procedures to personality and motivational differences. *Journal of Consulting and Clinical Psychology, 43*, 1–8.

Billings, J.S. (1891). Vital statistics of the Jews. *New American Review, 153*, 70–84.

Birnbaum, A. (1991). Haven hugs and bugs. *American Journal of Hospice and Palliative Care, 8*, 23–29.

Blaxter, M. (1983). The causes of disease: Women talking. *Social Science & Medicine, 17*, 59–69.

Blaxter, M. (1985). Self-definition of health status and consulting rates in primary care. *Quarterly Journal of Social Affairs, 1*, 131–171.

Blaxter, M. (1995a). *Health and lifestyles*. London: Routledge.

Blaxter, M. (1995b). What is health? In B. Davey, A. Gray & C. Seale (Eds.), *Health and disease: A reader*. Buckingham and Philadelphia: Open University Press.

Blaxter, M. & Paterson, E. (1982). *Mothers and daughters: A three-generational study of health attitudes and behaviour*. London: Heinnemann.

Blazer, D.G. (1982). Social support and mortality in an elderly community population. *American Journal of Epidemiology, 115*, 684–694.

Bloor, M. & Horobin, G. (1975). Conflict and conflict resolution in doctor-patient relationships. In C. Cox and A. Mead (Eds.), *A sociology of medical practice* (pp. 271–284). London: Collier Macmillan.

Bourdieu, P. (1986). The forms of capital. In J. Richardson (Ed.), *Handbook of theory and research for the sociology of education* (pp. 241–258). New York: Macmillan.

Bowling, A. (1997). *Measuring health: A review of quality of life measurement scales, 2nd edn*. Buckingham and Philadelphia: Open University Press.

Bradley, C. (1985). Psychological aspects of diabetes. In D.G.M.M. Alberti and L.P. Drall (Eds.), *Diabetes Annual*. Amsterdam: Elsevier.

British Broadcasting Corporation/Health Education Authority (1990). *Quit and win*. London: BBC/HEA.

Bronfenbrenner, U. (1979). *The ecology of human development*. Cambridge, MA: Harvard University Press.

Bryson, L. & Mowbray, M. (1981). 'Community' – the spray-on solution. *Australian Journal of Social Issues, 16*, 255–267.

Budd, R.J. (1987). Response bias and the theory of reasoned action. *Social Cognition, 5*, 95–107.

Budd, R.J. & Spencer, C.P. (1985). Exploring the role of personal normative beliefs in the theory of reasoned action: The problem of discriminating between alternative path models. *European Journal of Social Psychology, 15*, 299–313.

Burnkrant, R.E. & Page, T.J. (1988). The structure and antecedents of the normative and attitudinal components of Fishbein's theory of reasoned action. *Journal of Experimental Social Psychology, 24*, 66–87.

Bury, M. (1997). *Health and illness in a changing society*. London: Routledge.

Busfield, J. (2000). *Health and health care in modern Britain*. Oxford: Oxford University Press.

Bush, R., Dower, J. & Mutch, A. (2002). *Community Capacity Index*. Centre for Primary Health Care, University of Queensland, Brisbane.

Byrd, R.C. (1988). Positive therapeutic effects of intercessory prayer in a coronary care unit population. *Southern Medical Journal, 81*, 826–829.

Calnan, M. (1984). The health belief model and participation in programmes for the early detection of breast cancer: A comparative analysis. *Social Science & Medicine, 19*, 823–830.

Calnan, M. (1987). *Health and illness: The lay perspective*. London: Tavistock.

Campbell, E.J.M., Scadding, J.G. & Roberts, R.S. (1979). The concept of disease. *British Medical Journal, 2*, 757–62.

Cancer Research Campaign/Teacher's Advisory Council on Alcohol and Drug Education (1988). *Packing it in*? Manchester: CRC/TACADE.

Casel, J.C. (1976). The contribution of the social environment to host resistance. *American Journal of Epidemiology, 104*, 107–123.

Charng, H.-W., Piliavin, J.A. & Callero, P.L. (1988). Role identity and reasoned action in the prediction of repeated behaviour. *Social Psychology Quarterly, 51*, 303–317.

Chassin, L., Presson, C.C., Sherman, S.J., Corty, E. & Olshavsky, R.W. (1984). Predicting the onset of cigarette smoking in adolescents: A longitudinal study. *Journal of Applied Social Psychology, 14*, 224–243.

Cimprich, B. (1993). Development of an intervention to restore attention in cancer patients. *Cancer Nursing, 16*, 83–92.

Clarke, M. & Kurinczuk, J.J. (1992). Health services research: A case of need or special pleading. *British Medical Journal, 304*, 1675–1676.

Clarke, R., Frost, C., Collins, R., Appleby, P. & Peto, R. (1997). Dietary lipids and blood cholesterol: Quantitative meta-analysis of metabolic ward studies. *British Medical Journal, 314*, 112–117.

Coan, R.W. (1973). Personality variables associated with cigarette smoking. *Journal of Personality and Social Psychology, 26*, 86–104.

Cockerham, W.C. (1999). *Health and social change in Russia and Eastern Europe*. London: Routledge.

Cockerham, W.C. (2001). *Medical sociology* (8th edn). Upper Saddle River, NJ: Prentice Hall.

Coggon, D., Rose, G. & Barker, D.J.P. (1993). *Epidemiology for the uninitiated* (3rd edn). London: BMJ Publishing Group.

Cohen, S. (1988). Psychosocial models of the role of social support in the etiology of physical disease. *Health Psychology, 7*, 269–297.

Coleman, J.S. (1990). *Foundations of Social Theory*. Cambridge, MA: Belknap Press of Harvard University Press.

Comstock, G.W. & Partridge, K.B. (1972). Church attendance and health. *Journal of Chronic Diseases, 25*, 665–672.

Cooper, J. & Croyle, R. (1984). Attitudes and attitude change. *Annual Review of Psychology, 35*, 395–426.

Cornwell, J. (1984). *Hard-earned lives: Accounts of health and illness from East London*. London: Tavistock Press.

Courtenay, W.H. (2000). Constructions of masculinity and their influence on men's well-being: A theory of gender and health. *Social Science & Medicine, 50*, 1385–1401.

Csikszentmihalyi, M. (1990). *Flow: The psychology of optimal experience*. New York: Harper and Row.

Csikszentmihalyi, M. (1993). Activity and happiness: Towards a science of occupation. *Journal of Occupational Science: Australia, 1*, 38–42.

Csikszentmihalyi, M. & LeFevre, J. (1989). Optimal experience in work and leisure. *Journal of Personality and Social Psychology, 56*, 5–22.

Cummings, K.M., Jette, A.M. & Brock, B.M. (1979). Psychosocial determinants of immunization behavior in a swine influenza campaign. *Medical Care, 17*, 639–649.

d'Houtard, A. & Field, M.G. (1984). The image of health: Variations in perception by social class in a French population. *Sociology of Health & Illness, 6*, 30–60.

Dahlin, L., Cederblad, M., Antonovsky, A. & Hagnell, O. (1990). Childhood vulnerability and adult invincibility. *Acta Psychiatry Scandanavia, 82*, 228–232.

Davidson, W.B. & Cotter, P.R. (1986). Measurement of sense of community within the sphere of the city. *Journal of Applied Social Psychology, 16*, 608–619.

Davis-Berman, J. & Berman, D.S. (1989). The wilderness therapy program: An empirical study of its effects with adolescents in an outpatient setting. *Journal of Contemporary Psychotherapy, 19*, 271–281.

Davison, C., Davey Smith, G. & Frankel, S. (1991). Lay epidemiology and the prevention paradox: The implications of coronary candidacy for health education. *Sociology of Health and Illness, 13*, 1–19.

DISC (1995). Efficacy and safety of lowering dietary intake of fat and cholesterol in children with elevated low-density lipoprotein cholesterol: The dietary intervention study in children (DISC). *Journal of the American Medical Association, 273*, 1429–1436.

Doherty, W.J. & Allen, W. (1994). Family functioning and parental smoking as predictors of adolescent cigarette use: A six-year prospective study. *Journal of Family Psychology, 8*, 347–353.

Downie, R.S., Tannahill, C. & Tannahill, A. (1996). *Health promotion models and values, 2nd edn.* Oxford: Oxford University Press.

Doyal, L. (2000). Gender equity in health. *Social Science & Medicine, 51,* 931–939.

Doyal, L. (2001). Sex, gender and health: The need for a new approach. *British Medical Journal, 323,* 1061–1063.

Draper, P., Griffiths, J., Dennis, J. & Popay, J. (1980). Three types of health education. *British Medical Journal, 281,* 493–495.

Draper, R.J., Gerber, G.J. & Layng, E.M. (1990). Defining the role of pet animals in psychotherapy. *Psychology Journal of the University of Ottowa, 15,* 169–172.

Dreon, D.M., Fernstrom, H.A., Miller, B. & Krauss, R.M. (1994). Low-density lipoprotein subclass patterns and lipoprotein response to a reduced-fat diet in men. *FASEB Journal, 8,* 121–126.

Durkheim, E. (1897). *La Suicide.* Paris: Alcan.

Eaton, L. (1999). Unknown quantities. *Health Service Journal,* 22 May.

Eberstadt, N. (1999). Russia: Too sick to matter? *Policy Review, 95,* 3–24.

Eckerman, L. (2000). Gendering indicators of health and well-being: Is quality of life gender-neutral? *Social Indicators Research, 52,* 29–54.

Edwards, W. (1954). The theory of decision-making. *Psychological Bulletin, 51,* 380–417.

Elo, I.T. & Preston, S.H. (1996). Educational differential in mortality: United States, 1979–85. *Social Science & Medicine, 42,* 47–57.

Emlen, S.T. (1997). The evolutionary study of human family systems. *Social Science Information, 36,* 563–589.

Emslie, C., Hunt, K. & Macintyre, S. (1999). Problematizing gender, work and health: The relationship between gender, occupational grade, working conditions and minor morbidity in full-time bank employees. *Social Science & Medicine, 48,* 33–48.

Ermisch, J. & Francesconi, M. (2000). The increasing complexity of family relationships: Lifetime experience of lone motherhood and stepfamilies in Great Britain. *European Journal of Population, 16,* 235–249.

Eskin, F. (1999). Response to Maynard. *Health Service Journal,* 24 June.

Evaluation of two school education programmes under normal classroom conditions. *British Medical Journal, 306,* 102–107.

Ewles, L. & Simnett, I. (1985). *Promoting health: A practical guide to health education.* Chichester: Wiley.

Fallowfield, L. (1990). *The quality of life: The missing measurement in health care.* London: Souvenir.

Farkas, A.J., Pierce, J.P., Zhu, S.-H., Rosbrook, B., Gilpin, E.A., Berry, C. & Kaplan, R.M. (1996). Addiction versus stages of change models in predicting smoking cessation. *Addiction, 91,* 1271–1280.

Fee, E. & Acheson, R.M. (Eds.) (1991). *A history of education in public health.* Oxford: Oxford University Press.

Fishbein, M. & Ajzen, I. (1975). *Belief, attitude, intention and behavior. An introduction to theory and research.* Reading, MA: Addison-Wesley.

Førde, O.H. (1998). Is imposing risk awareness cultural imperialism? *Social Science & Medicine, 47,* 1155–1159.

Foucault, M. (1973). *The birth of the clinic* (trans. A.M. Sheridan Smith). London: Tavistock.

Fox, N. (1998). Postmodernism and 'health'. In A. Petersen & C. Waddell (Eds.), *Health matters: A sociology of illness, prevention and care.* Buckingham: Open University Press.

Freidson, E. (1970). *Profession of medicine: A study of the sociology of applied knowledge.* New York: Harper Row.

Friedman, E. & Thomas, S.A. (1995). Pet ownership, social support, and one-year survival after acute myocardial infarction in the cardiac arrhythmia suppression trial. *American Journal of Cardiology, 76,* 1213–1217.

Frith, C.D. (1971). Smoking behaviour and its relation to the smoker's immediate experience. *British Journal of Social and Clinical Psychology, 10*, 73–78.

Frumkin, H. (2001). Beyond toxicity: Human health and the natural environment. *American Journal of Preventive Medicine, 20*, 234–240.

Fuhrer, R., Stanfield, S.A., Chemali, J. & Shipley, M.J. (1999). Gender, social relations and mental health: Prospective finding from an occupational cohort (Whitehall II Study). *Social Science & Medicine, 48*, 77–87.

Ghate, D. & Hazel, N. (2002). *Parenting in poor environments: Stress, support and coping.* London and Philadelphia: Jessica Kingsley.

Giddens, A. (1990). *The consequences of modernity.* Cambridge: Polity Press.

Giddens, A. (1991). *Modernity and self-identity: Self and society in the late modern age.* Cambridge: Polity Press.

Ginn, J. & Arber, S. (1999). Women's pension poverty: Prospects and options for change (pp. 75–97). In S. Walby (Ed.), *New agendas for women.* London: Macmillan.

Good, B.J. (1994). *Medicine, rationality and experience: An anthropological perspective.* Cambridge: Cambridge University Press.

Goodman, E. (2002). How much does socioeconomic status matter to adolescent health? *Journal of Adolescent Health, 30*, 102.

Goodman, E., Amick, B.C., Rezendes, M.O., Levine, S., Kagan, J., Rogers, W.H. & Tarlov, A.R. (2000). Adolescents' understanding of social class: A comparison of white upper middle class and working class youth. *Journal of Adolescent Health, 27*, 80–83.

Green, G., Macintyre, S., West, P. & Ecob, R. (1990). Do children of lone parents smoke more because their mothers do? *British Journal of Addiction, 86*, 745–758.

Griffiths, S. (1999). Response to Maynard. *Health Service Journal*, 24 June.

Habermas, J. (1970). On symbolically distorted communication and towards a theory of communicative competence. *Inquiry, 13*, 2205–2218 and 360–375.

Hadden, F. (1999). Non-medical worthies would not necessarily be more cost-effective. *Health Science Journal*, 24th June.

Hall, H. (1910). The work cure. *Boston Medical and Surgical Journal, 54*, 13–15.

Hardey, M. (1998). *The social context of health.* Buckingham and Philadelphia, PA: Open University Press.

Hartig, T., Mang, M. & Evans, G. (1991). Restorative effects of natural environmental experiences. *Environment and Behaviour, 23*, 3–26.

Hawe, P. & Shiell, A. (2000). Social capital and health promotion: A review. *Social Science & Medicine, 51*, 871–885.

Hawe, P., King, L., Noort, M., Jordens, C. & Lloyd, B. (2000). *Indicators to help with capacity-building in health promotion.* New South Wales: Health Department.

Health Development Agency (2004). www.hda-online.org.uk

Health Education Authority (1989). *How to Stop Smoking for You and Your Baby.* HEA.

Health Education Authority (1990a). *A Smoker's Guide to Giving Up.* HEA.

Health Education Authority (1990b). *Family Smoking Education Project, Pupil's Booklet.* HEA.

Health Education Authority (1997). Personal communication.

Health Education Authority/British Broadcasting Corporation (1990). *Quit and Win!*

Health Education Board for Scotland (1998). *So you want to cut down your drinking? A self-help guide to sensible drinking.* Edinburgh: HEBS.

Health of the nation: A strategy for health in England (1992). London: HMSO.

Health Education Council (1986). Women and smoking: A guide for action. London: HEC.

Health of the Nation, The (1992). *A strategy for health in England.* London: HMSO.

Heerwagen, J.H. (1990). The psychological aspects of windows and window design. In K.H. Anthony, J. Choi & B. Orland (Eds.), *Proceedings of the 21st Annual Conference of the Environmental Research Association* (pp. 269–280). Oklahoma City: EDRA.

Heider, F. (1944). Social perception and phenomenal causality. *Psychological Review, 51*, 358–374.

Heider, F. (1958). *The psychology of interpersonal relations*. New York: John Wiley.

Herrnstein, R.J. & Murray, C. (1994). *The bell shaped curve: Intelligence and class structure in American life*. London: Free Press.

Hertzman, C. (1995). *Environment and health in Eastern and Central Europe*. Washington, DC: World Bank.

Herzlich, C. (1973). *Health and illness: A social psychological analysis*. London: Academic Press.

Hill, A.B. (1965). The environment and disease: Association or causation? *Proceedings of the Royal Society of Medicine, 58*, 1217–1219.

Hobbs, T.R. & Shelton, G.C. (1972). Therapeutic camping for emotionally disturbed adolescents. *Hospital and Community Psychiatry, 23*, 298–301.

Holland, W. (2002). *Foundations for health improvement: Productive epidemiological public health research 1919–1998*. The Nuffield Trust for Research and Policy in Health Services. London: HMSO.

Holme, I. (1990). An analysis of randomised controlled trial evaluating the effect of cholesterol reduction on total mortality and coronary heart disease incidence. *Circulation, 82*, 1916–1924.

Honeyman, M.K. (1992). Vegetation and stress: A comparison study of varying amounts of vegetation in countryside and urban scenes. In D. Relf (Ed.), *The role of horticulture in human well-being and social development: A national symposium* (19–21 April, Arlington, Virginia) (pp. 143–145). Portland, OR: Timber Press.

House, J.S., Landis, K.R. & Umberson, D. (1988). Social relationships and health. *Science, 241*, 540–545.

Hull, R.B. & Revell, G.R.B. (1989). Cross-cultural comparison on landscape scenic beauty evaluations: A case study in Bali. *Journal of Environmental Psychology, 9*, 177–191.

Hunt, L.M. (1985). Relativism in the diagnosis of hypoglycemia. *Social Science & Medicine, 20*, 1289–1294.

Hunt, K. & Annandale, E. (1999). Relocating gender and morbidity: Examining men's and women's health in contemporary western societies. Introduction to special issue. *Gender & Health, 48*, 1–5.

Hyer, L., Boyd, S., Scurfield, R., Smith, D. & Burke, J. (1996). Effects of outward bound experience as an adjunct to inpatient PTSD treatment of war veterans. *Journal of Clinical Psychology, 52*, 263–278.

Ikard, F.F., Green, D.E. & Horn, D. (1969). A scale to differentiate between types of smoking as related to the management of affect. *International Journal of the Addictions, 4*, 649–659.

Illich, I. (1976). *The limits of medicine*. London: Marion Boyars.

Isohanni, M., Moilanen, I. & Rantakillo, P. (1991). Determinants of teenage smoking, with special reference to non-standard family background. *British Journal of Addiction, 86*, 391–398.

Jenkins, C.D. (1971). Psychologic and social precursors of coronary disease. *New England Journal of Medicine, 284*, 244–255, 307–317.

Jerstad, L. & Stelzer, J. (1973). Adventure experiences as treatment for residential mental patients. *Therapeutic Recreation Journal, 7*, 8–11.

Jung, C.G. (1928). Two essays on analytical psychology. *Complete Works 7*. London: Routledge & Kegan Paul.

Kalimo, R. & Vuori, J. (1990). Work and sense of coherence: Resources for competence and life satisfaction. *Behavioral Medicine, 16*, 76–89.

Kalimo, R. & Vuori, J. (1991). Work factors and health: The predictive role of pre-employment experiences. *Journal of Occupational Psychology, 64*, 97–115.

Karpf, A. (1988). *Doctoring the box.* London: Routledge.

Katcher, A., Segal, H. & Beck, A. (1984). Comparison of contemplation and hypnosis for the reduction of anxiety and discomfort during dental surgery. *American Journal of Clinical Hypnosis, 27,* 14–21.

Kellert, S.R. & Wilson, E.O. (1993). *The biophilia hypothesis.* Washington, DC: Island Press.

Kennedy, E. & Offutt, S. (2000). Alternative nutrition outcomes using a fiscal food policy. *British Medical Journal, 320,* 301–305.

Kennedy, E.T., Ohls, J., Carlson, S. & Fleming, K. (1999). The healthy eating index: Design and application. *Journal of the American Dietary Association, 95,* 1103–1108.

Keyes, A., Anderson, J. & Grande, R. (1965). Serum cholesterol response to changes in diet (IV). Particular fats in the diet. *Metabolism, 14,* 776–786.

King, H. & Locke, F.B. (1980). American White Protestant clergy as a low-risk population for mortality research. *Journal of the National Cancer Institute, 65,* 1115–1124.

King, J.B. (1982). The impact of patients' perceptions of high blood pressure on attendance at screening. *Social Science & Medicine, 16,* 1079–1092.

Knott, V.J. (1979). Personality, arousal and individual differences in cigarette smoking. *Psychological Reports, 45,* 423–428.

Kolata, G. (2001). Cancer screening faces rising scientific doubt. *International Herald Tribune,* 31 December 2001–1 January 2002, p. 2.

Korpela, K. & Hartig, T. (1996). Restorative qualities of favourite places. *Journal of Environmental Psychology, 16,* 221–233.

Laslett, P. (1989). *A fresh map of Life.* London: Weidenfeld and Nicolson.

Lau, R.R. (1995). Cognitive representations of health and illness. In D. Gochman (Ed.), *Handbook of Health Behaviour Research,* Vol. 1 (pp. 51–69). London, Thousand Oaks, CA and New Delhi: Sage.

Law, M.R., Wald, N.J. & Thompson, S.G. (1994). By how much and how quickly does reduction in serum cholesterol concentration lower risk of ischaemic heart disease? *British Medical Journal, 308,* 367–373.

Levin, J.S. (1994). Religion and health: Is there an association, is it valid, and is it causal? *Social Science & Medicine, 38,* 1475–1482.

Levin, J.S. & Schiller, P.L. (1987). Is there a religious factor in health? *Journal of Religion and Health, 26,* 9–36.

Levin, J.S. & Vanderpool, H.Y. (1989). Is frequent religious attendance really conducive to better health? Toward an epidemiology of religion. *Social Science & Medicine, 24,* 589–600.

Levine, D. (1994). Breaking through barriers: Wilderness therapy for sexual assault survivors. *Women and Therapy, 15,* 175–184.

Lewis, C.A. (1996). *Green nature/human nature: The meaning of plants in our lives.* Urbana, IL: University of Illinois Press.

Lloyd, B. & Lucas, K. (1997). *Why do adolescent girls smoke? A quantitative/behavioural study.* London: Department of Health.

Lloyd, B. & Lucas, K. (1998). *Smoking in adolescence: Images and identities.* London and New York: Routledge.

Lloyd, B., Lucas, K. & Fernbach, M. (1997). Adolescent girls' constructions of smoking identities: Implications for health promotion. *Journal of Adolescence, 20,* 43–56.

Lord, J. & Farlow, D.M. (1990). A study of personal empowerment: Implications for health promotion. *Health Promotion (Canada), 29,* 2–8.

Lucas, K. (1994). *The relationship between beliefs, attitudes, negative affect and changes in changes in smoking behaviour during pregnancy.* D.Phil. Thesis, University of Sussex, UK.

Lucas, K. & Lloyd, B. (1999). Starting smoking: Girls' explanations of the influence of peers. *Journal of Adolescence, 22,* 647–655.

Luck, G.M. & Luckman, J. (1974). *Patients, hospitals and operational research*. London: Tavistock.

Ludmerer, K.M. (1999). *Time to heal: American medical education from the turn of the century to the era of managed care*. Oxford: Oxford University Press.

Lundberg, O. & Nyström Peck, M. (1994). Sense of coherence, social structure and health. *European Journal of Public Health, 4*, 252–257.

Macintyre, S. (1993). Gender differences in the perceptions of common cold symptoms. *Social Science & Medicine, 36*, 15–20.

Macintyre, S., Ford, G. & Hunt, K. (1999). Do women 'over-report' morbidity? Men's and women's responses to structured prompting on a standard question on longstanding illness. *Social Science & Medicine, 48*, 89–98.

Maclaine, K. & MacLeod Clark, J. (1991). Womens' reasons for smoking in pregnancy. *Nursing Times, 87*, 22, 39–42.

Macleod, J., Smith, G.D., Heslop, P., Metcalfe, C., Carroll, D. & Hart, C. (2002). Psychological stress and cardiovascular disease: Empirical demonstration of bias in a prospective observational study of Scottish men. *British Journal of Medicine, 324*, 1247–1251.

Macleod Clark, J., Haverty, S. & Kendall, S. (1990). Helping people to stop smoking: A study of the nurse's role. *Journal of Advanced Nursing, 16*, 357–363.

MacMahon, B. & Trichopoulos, D. (1996). *Epidemiology: Principles and methods*. Boston: Little Brown & Company.

Maibach, E.W., Rothschild, M.L. & Novelli, W.D. (2002). Social marketing. In K. Glanz et al., *Health behavior and health education: Theory, research and practice*. San Francisco: Jossey Bass.

Maiman, L.A. & Becker, M.H. (1974). The health belief model: Origins and correlates in psychological theory. *Health Education Monographs, 2*, 336–358.

Manstead, A.S., Proffitt, C. & Smart, J.L. (1983). Predicting and understanding mothers' infant feeding intentions and behaviour: Testing the theory of reasoned action. *Journal of Personality and Social Psychology, 44*, 657–671.

Marmot, M. (1999). Introduction. In M. Marmot & R.G. Wilkinson (Eds.), *Social determinants of health*. Oxford and New York: Oxford University Press.

Marmot, M. & Wilkinson, R.G. (Eds.) (1999). *Social determinants of health*. Oxford and New York: Oxford University Press.

Marmot, M.G., Rose, G., Shipley, M. & Hamilton, P.J.S. (1978). Employment grade and coronary heart disease in British civil servants. *Epidemiology and Community Health, 32*, 244–249.

Marshall, T. (2000). Exploring a fiscal food policy: The case of diet and ischaemic heart disease. *British Medical Journal, 320*, 301–305.

Marx, J.D. (1988). An outdoor adventure counselling program for adolescents. *Social Work, 33*, 517–520.

Matthews, S., Manor, O. & Power, C. (1999). Social inequalities in health: Are there gender differences? *Social Science & Medicine, 48*, 49–60.

Maynard, A. (1999). Money down the drains. *Health Service Journal*, 10 June.

Mazel, D. (2000). *American literary environmentalism*. Athens, GA: University of Georgia Press.

McDonough, P. & Walters, V. (2001). Gender and health: Reassessing patterns and explanations. *Social Science & Medicine, 52*, 547–559.

McIntyre, K.O., Lichtenstein, E. & Marmelstein, R.J. (1983). Self-efficacy and relapse in smoking cessation: A replication and extension. *Journal of Consulting and Clinical Psychology, 51*, 632–633.

McKennell, A.C. (1970). Smoking motivation factor. *British Journal of Social and Clinical Psychology, 9*, 8–22.

McKennell, A.C. & Thomas, R.K. (1967). *Adults' and adolescents' smoking habits and attitudes.* London: HMSO.

McKeown, T. (1976). *The role of medicine: Dream, mirage or Nemesis?* London: Nuffield Provincial Hospitals Trust.

McKinley, J.B. (1972). Some approaches and problems in the study of the use of services – an overview. *Journal of Health and Social Behaviour, 13*, 115.

McLuhan, T.C. (1994). *The way of the Earth: Encounters with nature in ancient and contemporary thought.* New York: Simon and Schuster.

Meyer, A. (1922). The philosophy of occupational therapy. *Archives of Occupational Therapy, 1*, 1–10.

Michie, S., Marteau, T.M. & Kidd, J. (1990). Cognitive predictors of attendance at antenatal classes. *British Journal of Clinical Psychology, 29*, 193–199.

Michie, S. & Abraham, C. (2004). Interventions to change behaviours: Evidence-based or evidence-inspired? *Psychology and Health, 19*, 29–49.

Miniard, P. & Cohen, J.B. (1981). An examination of the Fishbein–Ajzen behavioral intentions model's concepts and measures. *Journal of Experimental Social Psychology, 17*, 309–339.

Mirowsky, J. (1999). Subjective life expectancy in the US: Correspondence to actuarial estimates by age, sex and race. *Social Science & Medicine, 49*, 967–979.

Moyer, J.A. (1988). Bannock bereavement retreat: A camping experience for surviving children. *American Journal of Hospice Care, 5*, 26–30.

Moynihan, R., Heath, I. & Henry, D. (2002). Selling sickness: The pharmaceutical industry and disease mongering. *British Journal of Medicine, 324*, 886–890.

Mullen, P.D., Hersey, J.C. & Iverson, D.C. (1987). Health models compared. *Social Science & Medicine, 16*, 323–331.

Murphy, P.D., Gifford, T. & Yamazato, K. (1998). *Literature of nature: An international sourcebook.* Chicago: Fitzroy Dearborn Publishers.

Myrsten, A.L., Anderssen, K., Frankenaeuser, M. & Elgerot, A. (1975). Immediate effects of cigarette smoking as related to different smoking habits. *Perceptual Motor Skills, 40*, 515–523.

Nash, R. (1982). *Wilderness and the American mind* (3rd edn). New Haven, CT: Yale University Press.

Nettleton, S. (1995). *The sociology of health and illness.* Cambridge and Malden, MA: Polity Press.

North, D.C. (1990). *Institutions, institutional change and economic performance.* New York: Cambridge University Press.

Nutbeam, D. (1986). Health promotion glossary. *Health Promotion, 1*, 113–126.

Nutbeam, D. & Harris, E. (2004). *Theory in a nutshell* (2nd edn). New York: McGraw-Hill.

Nutbeam, D., Macaskill, P., Smith, C., Simpson, J.M. & Catford, J. (1993). Evaluation of two school education programmes under normal classroom conditions. *British Medical Journal, 306*, 102–107.

O'Connor, K. (1985). A model of situational preference among smokers. *Personality and Individual Differences, 6*, 151–160.

O'Neill, R. (2002). *Experiments in living: The fatherless family.* London: www.civitas.org.uk.

Oakley, A. (1980). *Women confined: Towards a sociology of childbirth.* Oxford: Martin Robertson.

Office for National Statistics (2001). *Mortality statistics: General review of the Registrar General on Death in England and Wales.* DH1, Series 32.

Office of National Statistics (2001). *Accommodation type: By household composition.* Social Trends, 34. London: ONS.

Office of National Statistics (2004). *Expectation of life (in years) at birth and selected age, 1981 onwards.* Health Statistics Quarterly, 26. London: ONS.

Ogden, J. (1996). *Health psychology: A textbook.* Buckingham and Philadelphia: Open University Press.

Oliver, R. & Berger, P. (1979). A path analysis of preventive health care decision models. *Journal of Consumer Research, 6,* 113–122.

Paisley, C.M. & Sparks, P. (1998). Expectations of reducing fat intake: The role of perceived need within the Theory of Planned Behaviour. *Psychology and Health, 13,* 341–353.

Palmer, M. (1997). *Freud and Jung on religion.* London and New York: Routledge.

Parsons, T. (1951). *The social system.* Glencoe, IL: The Free Press.

Parsons, T. (1972). Definitions of health and illness in the light of American values and social structure. In E. Jaco & E. Gartley (Eds.), *Patients, physicians and illness: A sourcebook in behavioural science and health* (pp. 165–187). London: Collier-Macmillan.

Pearse, I.H. & Crocker, L.H. (1943). *The Peckham Experiment: A study in the living structure of society.* London: Allen and Unwin.

Pearson, J. (1989). A wilderness program for adolescents with cancer. *Journal of the Association of Pediatric Oncology Nurses, 6,* 24–25.

Pederson, L.L., Wanklin, J.M. & Baskerville, J.C. (1984). The role of health beliefs in compliance with physician advice to quit smoking. *Social Science & Medicine, 19,* 573–580.

Pierce, J.P., Farkas, A., Zhu, S.-H., Berry, C. & Kaplan, R.M. (1996). Should the stage of change model be challenged? *Addiction, 91,* 1290–1292.

Pill, R. & Stott, N. (1982). Concepts of illness causation and responsibility: Some preliminary data from a sample of working class mothers. *Social Science & Medicine, 16,* 13–51.

Plakun, E.M., Tucker, G.J. & Harris, P.Q. (1981). Outward bound: An adjunctive psychiatric therapy. *Journal of Psychiatric Treatment Evaluation, 3,* 33–37.

Porter, R. (1995). Medical science and human science in the enlightenment. In C. Fox & R. Porter (Eds.), *Inventing human science: Eighteenth-century domains* (pp. 53–87). Berkeley: University of California Press.

Portes, A. (1998). *Social capital: Its origins and applications.* New York: Russell Sage.

Prior, L. (2000). Reflections on the 'mortal' body in late modernity. In S.J. Williams, J. Gabe & M. Calnan (Eds.), *Health, medicine and society: Key theories, future agendas* (pp. 186–202). London and New York: Routledge.

Prochaska, J.O. (1979). *Systems of psychotherapy: A transtheoretical analysis.* Homewood, IL: Dorsey Press.

Prochaska, J.O. & DiClemente, C.C. (1982a). Transtheoretical therapy: Toward a more integrative model of change. *Psychotherapy: Theory, Research and Practice, 19,* 276–288.

Prochaska, J.O. & DiClemente, C.C. (1982b). Self-change processes, self-efficacy and self-concept in relapse and maintenance of smoking. *Psychological Reports, 51,* 983–990.

Prochaska, J.O. & DiClemente, C.C. (1983). Stages and processes of self-change of smoking: Toward an integrative model of change. *Journal of Consulting and Clinical Psychology, 51,* 390–395.

Purcell, A.T., Lamb, R.J., Peron, E.M. & Falchero, S. (1994). Preference or preferences for landscape? *Journal of Environmental Psychology, 14,* 195–209.

Putnam, R.D. (1993). *Making democracy work: Civic transitions in modern Italy.* Princeton, NJ: Princeton University Press.

Putnam, R.D. (1995). Bowling alone: America's declining social capital. *Journal of Democracy, 6,* 65–78.

Putnam, R.D. (1997). Democracy in America at century's end. In A. Hardenius (Ed.), *Democracy's victory and crisis* (pp. 27–70). New York: Cambridge University Press.

Pybus, M.W. & Thomson, M.C. (1985). Health awareness and health actions of parents (ANZERCH/APHA conference 1979). In J. Boddy (Ed.), *Health: Perspectives and practice* (pp. 9–22). New Zealand: The Dunmore Press.

Raeburn, J. & Rootman, I. (1998). *People centred health promotion*. Chichester: John Wiley and Sons.

Rappaport, J. (1981). In praise of paradox: A social policy of empowerment over prevention. *American Journal of Community Psychology, 9*, 1–25.

Reilly, M.A. (1966). A psychiatric occupational therapy program as a teaching model. *American Journal of Occupational Therapy, 22*, 61.

Riley, J.N. (1977). Western medicine's attempt to become more scientific: Examples from the United States and Thailand. *Social Science & Medicine, 11*, 549.

Roberts, R., Towell, T. & Golding, J.F. (2001). *Foundations of health psychology*. London: Palgrave.

Rogers, E.M. (1983). *Diffusion of innovations*. Glencoe, IL: Free Press.

Rogers, E.M. (2002). Diffusion of preventative interventions. *Addictive Behaviours, 27*, 989–993.

Rose, R. (2000). How much does social capital add to individual health? A survey of Russians. *Social Science & Medicine, 51*, 1421–1435.

Rosenstock, I.M. (1966). Why people use health services. *Milbank Memorial Fund Quarterly, 44*, 94–124.

Rosenstock, I.M. (1974). The health belief model and preventive health behaviour. *Health Education Monographs, 2*, 354–386.

Ross, C.E. & Bird, C.E. (1994). Sex stratification and health life-style: Consequences for men's and women's perceived health. *Journal of Health and Social Behaviour, 35*, 161–178.

Rothman, J. (2001). Approaches to community interventions. In J. Rothman, J.L. Erlich & J.E. Tropman (Eds.), *Strategies of community interventions*. Hascam, IL: Peacock Publishers.

Rothstein, W.G. (2001). Trends in mortality in the twentieth century. In D.A. Matcha (Ed.), *Readings in medical sociology* (pp. 53–70). London: Allyn and Bacon.

Royal College of Physicians (2004). *Storing up problems: The medical case for a slimmer nation*. London: RCP.

Russell, M.A.H., Peto, J. & Patel, V.A. (1974). The classification of smoking by factorial structure of motives. *Journal of the Royal Statistical Society, Series A*, 313–346.

Rutter, D.R. & Bunce, D.J. (1989). The theory of reasoned action of Fishbein and Ajzen: A test of Touriss' amended procedure for measuring beliefs. *British Journal of Social Psychology, 28*, 39–46.

Sacks, O. (1984). *A leg to stand on*. New York: Harper-Collins.

Salovey, P. & Rothman, A.J. (2003). *Social psychology of health: Key Readings*. New York and Hove: Psychology Press.

Sarason, S.B. (1974). *A psychological sense of community: Prospects for a community psychology*. San Francisco: Jossey Bass.

Schalling, D. (1977). Personality and situational determinants of smoking: An example of interaction. In D. Magusson & N.S. Endler (Eds.), *Personality at the crossroads: Current issues in international psychology*. Hillsdale, NJ: Erlbaum.

Schlegel, R.P., Crawford, C.A. & Sanborn, M.D. (1977). Correspondence and mediational properties of the Fishbein model: An application to adolescent alcohol use. *Journal of Experimental Social Psychology, 13*, 421–430.

Seedhouse, D. (1986). *Health: The Foundations for achievement*. Chichester: John Wiley.

Serpell, J. (1991). Beneficial effects of pet ownership on some aspects of human health and behaviour. *Journal of the Royal Society of Medicine, 84*, 717–720.

Siegel, J. (1990). Stressful life events and use of physician services among the elderly: The moderation role of pet ownership. *Journal of Personality and Social Psychology, 58,* 1081–1086.

Sherman, S.J., Presson, C.C., Chassin, L., Bensenberg, M., Corty, E. & Olshavsky, R.W. (1982). Smoking intentions in adolescents: Direct experience and predictability. *Personality and Social Psychology Bulletin, 8,* 376–383.

Skolbekken, J.-A. (1995). The risk epidemic in medical journals. *Social Science & Medicine, 40,* 291–305.

Skrabanek, P. & McCormick, J. (1990). *Follies and fallacies in medicine.* New York: Prometheus Books.

Smith, R. (2002). In search of 'non-disease'. *British Journal of Medicine, 324,* 883–885.

Stockwell, T. (1996). Interventions cannot ignore intentions. *Addiction, 91,* 1283–1284.

Sutton, S.R. (1987). Social-psychological approaches to understanding addictive behaviours: Attitude-behaviour and decision-making models. *British Journal of Addiction, 82,* 355–370.

Sutton, S.R. (1989). Smoking attitudes and behaviour: Applications of Fishbein and Ajzen's theory of reasoned action to predicting and understanding smoking decisions. In T. Ney & A. Gale (Eds.), *Smoking and human behaviour* (pp. 289–312). London: John Wiley & Sons.

Sutton, S.R. (1996). Further support for the stages of change model? *Addiction, 91,* 1287–1289.

Sutton, S.R. & Eiser, J.R. (1984). The effect of fear-arousing communications on cigarette smoking: An expectancy-value approach. *Journal of Behavioral Medicine, 7,* 13–33.

Sutton, S.R., Marsh, A. & Matheson, J. (1987). Explaining smokers' decisions to stop: An expectancy-value approach. *Social Behaviour, 2,* 35–49.

TACADE/Health Education Council (1984). *Schools Health Education Project.* London: HEC.

Tang, J.L., Armitage, J.M., Lancaster, T., Silagy, C.A., Fowler, G.H. & Neil, H.A.W. (1998). Systematic review of dietary intervention trials to lower blood total cholesterol in free-living subjects. *British Medical Journal, 316,* 1213–1220.

Tannahill, A. (1985). What is health promotion? *Health Education Journal, 44,* 167–168.

Tarlov, A.R. (1996). Social determinant of health: The sociobiological translation. In D. Blane, E. Brunner & R. Wilkinson (Eds.), *Health and social organization: Towards a health policy for the 21st Century.* London: Routledge.

Taylor, W.C., Pass, T.M., Shepard, D.S. & Komaroff, A.L. (1987). Cholesterol reduction and life expectancy: A model incorporating multiple risk factors. *Annals of Internal Medicine, 106,* 605–614.

Tennessen, C.M. & Cimprich, B. (1995). Views to nature: Effects on attention. *Journal of Environmental Psychology, 15,* 77–85.

Tomkins, S.S. (1966). Psychological model for smoking behavior. *American Journal of Public Health, 12,* 17–20.

Tomkins, S.S. (1968). A modified model of smoking behavior. In E.F. Borgatta & R.P. Evans (Eds.), *Smoking, health and behavior.* Chicago, IL: Aldine.

Tones, K. & Tilford, S. (2001). *Health promotion: Effectiveness, efficiency and equity.* Cheltenham: Nelson Thornes.

Townsend, P., Davidson, N. & Whitehead, M. (1988). *Inequalities in health: The Black Report and the Health Divide.* Harmondsworth: Penguin.

Tudor, K. (1996). *Mental health promotion: Paradigms and practice.* London: Routledge.

Ulrich, R.S. (1984). View through a window may influence recovery from surgery. *Science, 224,* 420–421.

Ulrich, R.S. (1993). Biophilia, biophobia, and natural landscapes. In S.R. Kellert & E.O. Wilson (Eds.), *The biophilia hypothesis.* Washington, DC: Island Press.

Underwood, M.J. & Bailey, J.S. (1993). Should smokers be offered coronary bypass surgery? *British Medical Journal, 306,* 1047–1050.

Unwin, N., Carr, S. & Leeson, J. (1997). *An introductory study guide to public health and epidemiology.* Buckingham and Philadelphia: Open University Press.

Van den Burghe, P.L. (1989). Sociobiology. In A. Kuper and J. Kuper (Eds.), *The social science encyclopaedia* (pp. 795–798). London: Routledge.

Verrall, J. (1990). Community care – who's to benefit? Unpublished paper, available from Greenwich Welfare Rights Unit, Riverside House, Beresford Street, London SE18, UK.

Waitzkin, H. (1979). Medicine, superstructure and micropolitics. *Social Science & Medicine, 13,* 601–609.

Wallston, K.A. & Wallston, B.S. (1982). Who is responsible for your health? The construct of locus of control. In G.S. Sanders & J. Suls (Eds.), *Social Psychology of Health and Illness* (pp. 65–95). Hillsdale, NJ: Erlbaum.

Wallston, R.S. & Wallston, K.A. (1984). Social psychological models of health behaviour: An examination and integration. In A. Baum, S.E. Taylor & J.E. Singer (Eds.), *Handbook of psychology and health* (vol. 4, pp. 23–53). Hillsdale, NJ: Erlbaum.

Wanless, D. (2004). *Securing good health for the whole population. Final report,* February. London: The Stationery Office.

Warady, B.A. (1994). Therapeutic camping for children with end-stage renal disease. *Pediatric Nephrology, 8,* 387–390.

Warshaw, P.R. & Davis, F.D. (1985). Disentangling behavioural intention and behavioural expectation. *Journal of Experimental Social Psychology, 21,* 213–228.

Watson, P. (1995). Explaining rising mortality among men in Eastern Europe. *Social Science & Medicine, 41,* 923–934.

Weiss, C.H. (1979). The many meanings of research utilisation. *Public Health Review, 39,* 426–431.

West, P. (1997). Health inequalities in the early years: Is there equalisation in youth? *Social Science & Medicine, 30,* 665–673.

Wilcock, A. (1998). An occupational perspective of health. SLACK Incorporated, Australia.

Wilkinson, D. & Abraham, C. (2004). Constructing an integrated model of the antecedents of adolescent smoking. *British Journal of Health Psychology, 9,* 315–333.

Wilkinson, R.G. (1996). *Unhealthy societies: The afflictions of inequality.* London and New York: Routledge.

Wilkinson, R. & Marmot, M. (Eds.) (1998). *Social determinants of health: The solid facts.* New York: World Health Organization.

Williams, R. (1983). Concepts of health: An analysis of lay logic. *Sociology, 17,* 185–205.

Williams, S.J. & Calnan, M. (1996). The 'limits' of medicalization? Modern medicine and the lay populace in 'late' modernity. *Social Science & Medicine, 42,* 1609–1620.

Wilson, E.O. (1984). *The diversity of life.* Cambridge, MA: Harvard University Press.

Wilson, E.J.Q. (2002). *The marriage problem.* New York: Harper Collins.

Witman, J.P. (1987). The efficacy of adventure programming in the development of co-operation and trust with adolescents in treatment. *Therapeutic Recreation Journal, 21,* 22–29.

World Health Organization (1948). Constitution.

World Health Organization (1980). *International classification of impairments, Disabilities and handicaps.* Geneva: WHO.

World Health Organization (1992). *International classification of disease – 10.* Geneva: WHO.

World Health Organization (1994). *Progress towards health for all: Statistics of member states.* Geneva: WHO.

Yi, S.-L. (1985). A life renewed. *National Gardening, 8,* 19–21.

Author Index

Subject Index